Sensual Massage

A practical introduction

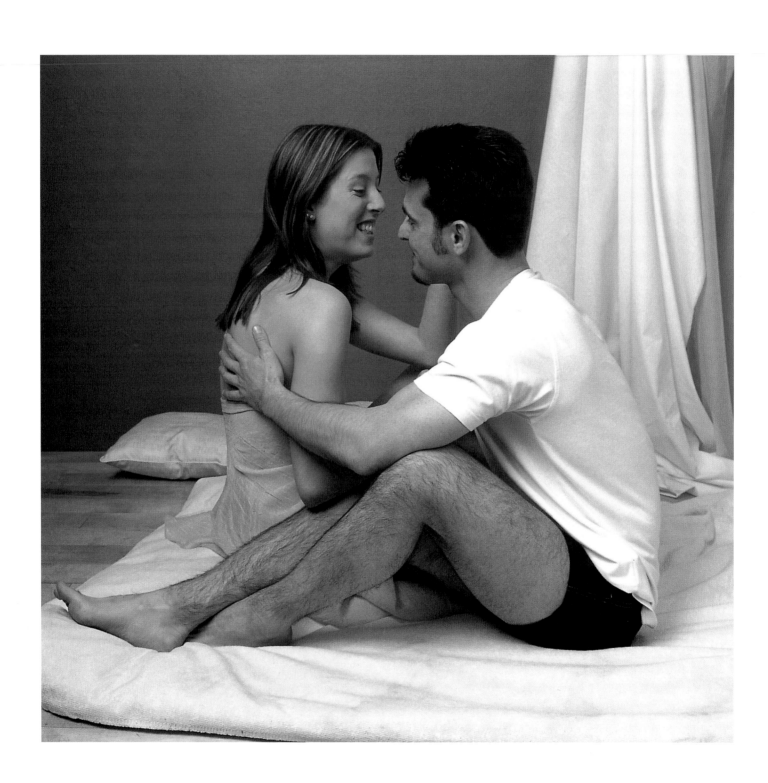

Sensual Massage

A practical introduction

DENISE WHICHELLO BROWN

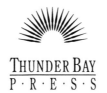

THUNDER BAY
P·R·E·S·S

Published in the United States by
Thunder Bay Press
5880 Oberlin Drive, Suite 400
San Diego, CA 92121-4794
http://wwww.advmkt.com

ISBN 1-57145-213-3

Library of Congress Cataloging-in Publication Data available upon request.

1 2 3 4 5 99 00 01 02 03

This book is not intended as a substitute for the advice of a health care professional. If you have any reason to believe you have a condition that affects your health, you must seek professional advice. Consult a qualified health care professional or your doctor before starting.

c o n t e n t s

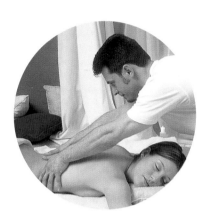

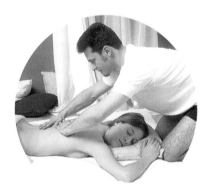

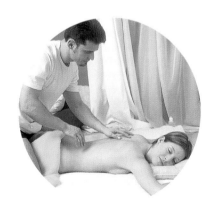

introduction to
Sensual Massage

BENEFITS OF SENSUAL MASSAGE

For thousands of years, lovers have delighted in the pleasures of sensual massage, and the joy of both giving and receiving pleasure from gentle touching and caressing has been recorded in cultures the world over. In today's climate of instant gratification, the art of sensual massage is equally important, giving lovers the chance to express their love in a tender and spiritual way.

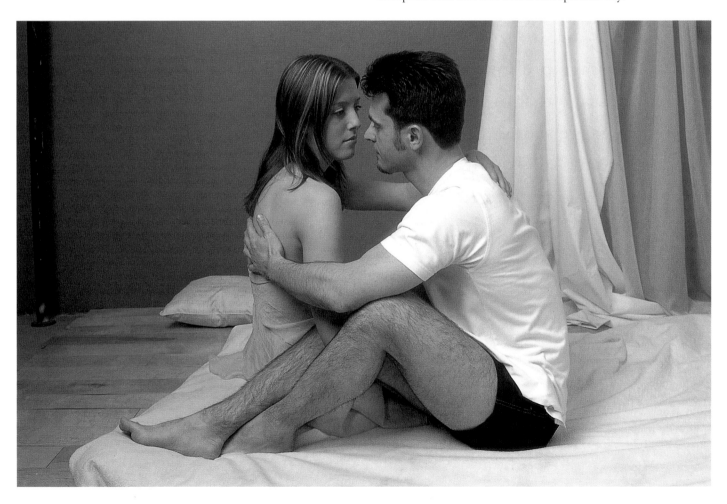

Sensual massage has been enjoyed by lovers all over the world for thousands of years.

The pleasures of sensual massage are described in the Indian Kama Sutra (meaning 'Scripture of Love'). Known primarily as an adventurous sex manual, the Kama Sutra also refers to the less explicit, but equally erotic, use of seductive oils and perfumes to heighten sensual pleasure.

In Egypt, sensual massage was common. Priests were skilled at making love potions and Egyptian women were well aware of how perfumes could be used for sexual attraction. In Greece we think of the goddess Aphrodite who was worshipped as the Goddess of Love, beauty and sexuality. It is of course from her name that the word 'aphrodisiac' is derived. From her son's name Eros comes the word 'erotic'. From Rome comes Venus the goddess of love and her son Cupid. The word 'venery' meaning sexual desire is derived from the word Venus. Public baths, which were visited by the Romans each day, were perfumed with rosewater, and fragrant oils were commonly rubbed into the body for sensual pleasure.

Josephine adored oils and employed them lavishly to tempt and seduce her lover Napoleon. A wide range of aromatic potions was used during their nights of passion.

All over the world since the dawn of civilization the use of massage coupled with sensual aromas to arouse sexual desire has been, and still is, widespread.

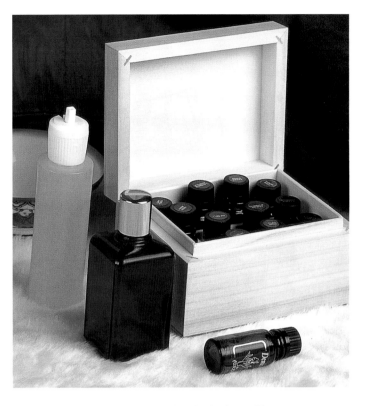

Massage using essential oils can provide a deeply pleasurable experience.

IMPORTANT NOTICE

This book must not be used as a substitute for treatment of medical conditions when it is important that the help of a doctor is sought. The information is not intended to diagnose or treat and any safety guidelines covered throughout the book must be adhered to.

It is of particular importance that essential oils are not to be taken internally and all other contra-indications regarding the oils are closely observed.

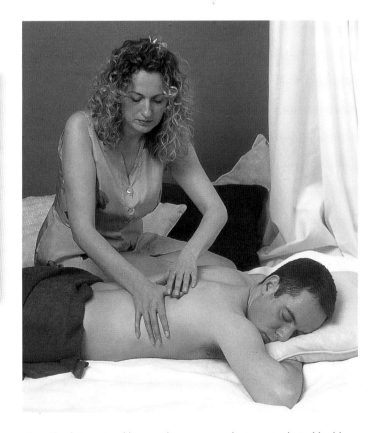

As well as being enjoyable, sensual massage can also promote physical health and a general sense of wellbeing.

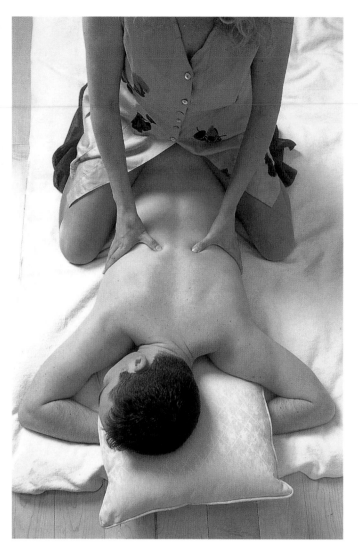

As well as being an exciting prelude to lovemaking, sensual massage can be equally enjoyable in itself. It is an excellent way of getting closer to your lover.

BENEFITS OF SENSUAL MASSAGE

The benefits of sensual massage have been known for a long time. It is not only one of the most pleasurable experiences imaginable, but will also strengthen the immune system thus improving your health and preventing disease from occurring.

Massage also stimulates our lymphatic system allowing the body to effectively eliminate toxins. It is also aids digestion, improving conditions such as constipation and irritable bowel syndrome, speeds up the circulation and improves breathing and bronchial disorders. Muscles are relaxed, alleviating neck, shoulder and back pain. Nerves are soothed and the stresses and strains of everyday life melt away.

Even when the act of sexual intercourse is not performed, the physical pleasure of touch in the form of sensual massage is extremely enjoyable. To both give and receive massage can be a highly sensual experience and can add a new dimension to your sex life.

In this book you will learn new and exciting techniques to bring more fun into your relationship with your lover. You will discover how to attract your lover and create your own exclusive love potions. As you enhance and harmonize your sexual relationships be assured that you are also helping to create and maintain a healthy and happy body.

Enjoy the sensual pleasures that lie before you!

getting Started

CREATING A SENSUAL AMBIENCE

It is essential to create a romantic and sensual environment for your massage, so try to prepare well in advance. Choose a time when you will not be disturbed. Take all telephones off the hook and do not allow children or pets to wander in and out of the room. Select some music, which you will both enjoy whether it be soothing and relaxing, or your own special piece.

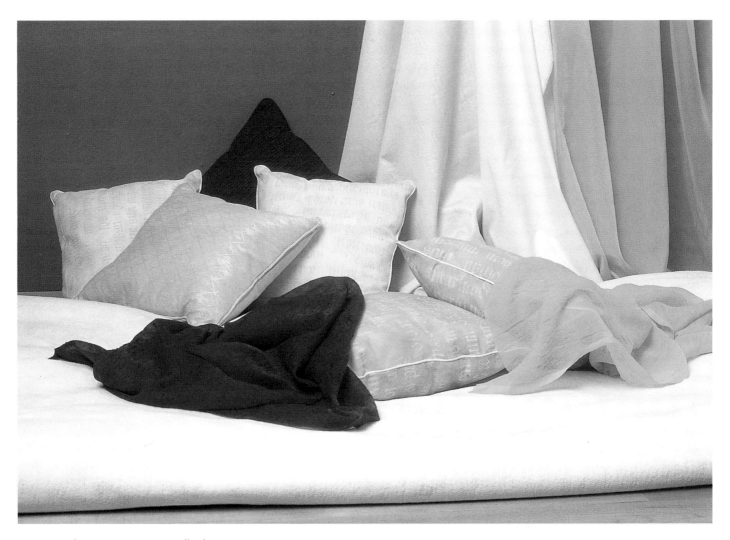

A warm and inviting environment will enhance your enjoyment of sensual massage.

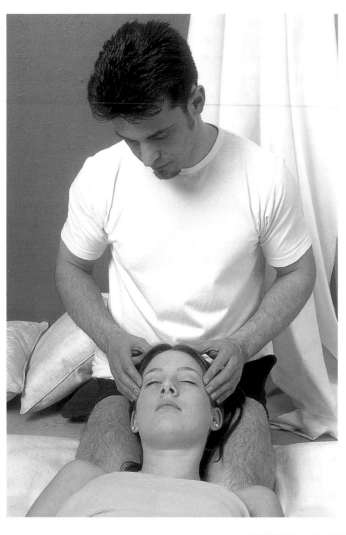

WARMTH

Heat the room beforehand to make it warm and inviting. If you are lucky enough to have an open fireplace, log fires are ideal. Your lover will find it is impossible to relax if he/she feels chilly, and the body temperature drops once the skin is exposed. Have plenty of throws, towels or blankets at your disposal to cover up any parts of the body that you are not working on. You will also need cushions or pillows, a small bowl and your massage oil on hand so that once you have started the massage you do not have to break contact with your lover.

LIGHTING

Lighting should be soft and romantic. Dim or turn off the lights and light a few candles around the room for the perfect setting. You may wish to use colored candles — pink candles will encourage romance and gentleness, red candles can induce passion and violet candles are deep and mysterious.

Softly flickering candles can heighten the sensual ambience of your room.

Make sure your lover is warm and relaxed. Provide plenty of throws and cushions, and remember not to break contact during the massage.

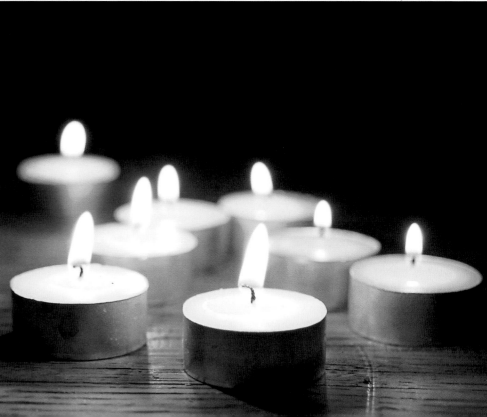

SCENTING

Scent the room by burning incense or even better use essential oils. A clay burner is perfect. Put a few teaspoons of water into the loose bowl on top and sprinkle a few drops of essential oil into it. Light the night-light and allow the wonderful aromas to diffuse into the atmosphere. You can achieve the same effect by putting a saucer or small bowl of warm water on top of a hot radiator and adding a few drops of essential oil to the water. Choose from any of the erotic oils outlined later in this book according to your aroma preference, or try one of the recipes below in your burner.

2 drops rose
2 drops sandalwood
OR
2 drops bergamot
2 drops neroli
OR
2 drops jasmine
2 drops geranium
OR
2 drops ylang ylang
2 drops rosewood

You may also decide to scent your towels,

pillows or bed linen. There are several ways of doing this:

*   Fill a small plant spray with spring water, add 10 drops of your chosen essential oil(s) and then spray your towels and pillows lightly.
*   Put a few drops of essential oil on to cotton-wool balls and place them inside your pillowcases or under your towels or sheets.
*   Add some drops of essential oil to the final rinse when washing your towels and pillowcases.

Particularly suitable oils would be frankincense, jasmine, neroli, patchouli, rose, sandalwood and ylang ylang as all these aromas have aphrodisiac properties and will last for a long time.

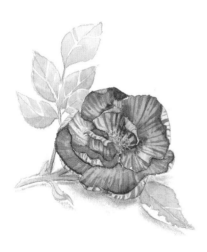

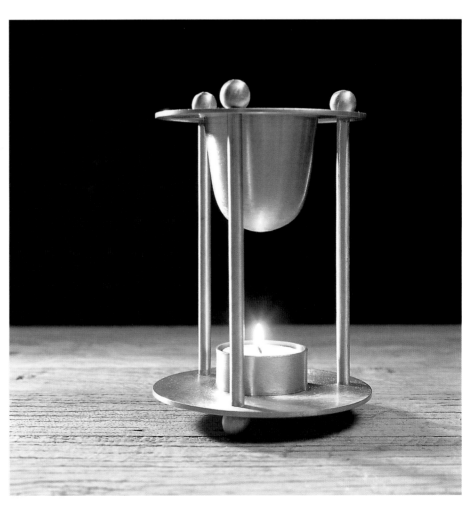

A few drops of your favourite oil in a burner or diffuser will give off a sensuous aroma.

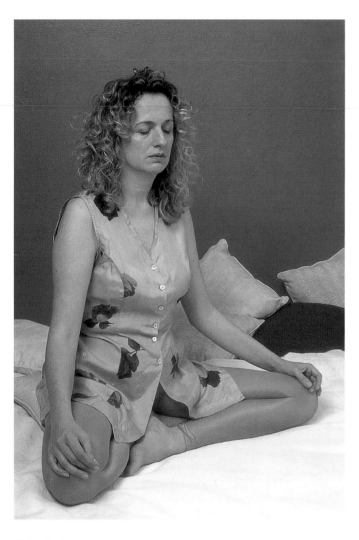

Before beginning your massage, it is important to centre yourself, to make sure you are completely relaxed.

CLOTHES

It is vital to wear comfortable and loose-fitting clothes preferably something short-sleeved or you will get too hot. You need to be able to move around your lover's body freely as you will often be changing your position. A loose T-shirt is ideal but any garments that are not constricting would be suitable. Go barefoot for maximum comfort and take off watches, bracelets, rings and necklaces which can scratch your lover's skin. Your lover should undress down to whatever level you both feel comfortable with. They should undress down to at least their underwear.

CENTERING YOURSELF

If you are to give a sensual massage a calm state of mind is essential. If you are feeling irritable, tired or depressed then your negative feelings will be transmitted to your lover. Therefore, prior to the massage you must try to completely empty your mind of your problems and spend time consciously relaxing yourself.

Lie down or sit comfortably with your back straight and take a few deep breaths from your abdomen allowing all your tension, mental and physical, to flow out of your body. If any thoughts pop into your head just let them go.

Stay in this relaxed position concentrating on your deep breathing for a few minutes until you feel completely relaxed. Breathe in peace and relaxation and as you breathe out let go of the tension from your mind and body.

MASSAGE SURFACE

Sensual massage can take place on a bed or on a firm well-padded surface. Spread out on the floor a thick duvet, two or three blankets, a sleeping bag or a futon. Use plenty of cushions or pillows to make your lover comfortable and relaxed during the massage.

When your lover is lying on his/her back place a cushion or pillow under the head and another one under the knees to take the pressure off the lower back. When your lover is lying on his/her front place a pillow or cushion under the shoulders one under the ankles and one under the abdomen if desired.

For your own comfort, and to avoid sore knees, make sure that you have something to kneel on too. You need to be just as relaxed as your lover.

Make sure your lover has plenty of cushions for comfort, otherwise the sensual atmosphere will be spoilt.

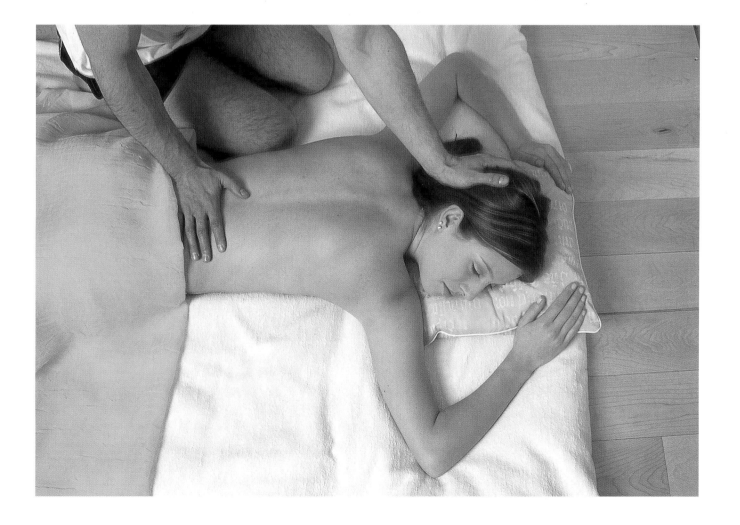

CONTRA-INDICATIONS

When Not to Massage

There are some occasions when you should not massage or need to take special care. If your partner has any of the following then wait until the condition has cleared up.

1. Fevers and high temperatures.
2. Skin infections, such as ringworm or scabies. Acne, psoriasis and eczema are not infectious.
3. Skin eruptions, open cuts and wounds — avoid the affected area.
4. Bruises — work around the bruise to help to disperse it.
5. Advanced varicose veins — do not work directly over them or you will cause further inflammation and pain.
6. Recent scar tissue (old scar tissue can be massaged).
7. Thrombosis or phlebitis — blood clots could be present and massage could move them with serious consequences.
8. Pregnancy — use only light movements over the abdomen during pregnancy.
9. Lumps and bumps — get these checked out by a doctor.

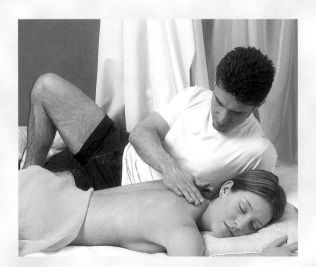
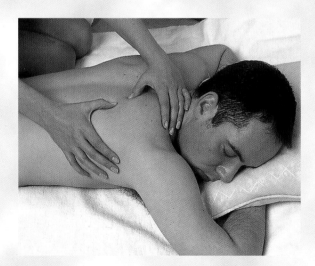

carrier
Oils

To enable your hands to glide smoothly and evenly over the contours of the body without jerkiness you will need carrier oil to work with. Your carrier oil (also known as a base or fixed oil) should be cold-pressed (i.e. not removed by heat), unrefined and additive-free. The base oil should be a vegetable, nut or seed oil. Such oils contain vitamins, minerals and fatty acids and therefore nourish the skin and are easily absorbed. Do not use mineral oil, such as baby oil, which is not easily absorbed and tends to clog the pores. Mineral oils lack the living quality of vegetable oils and can act as a barrier.

There is a wide variety of carrier oils available. The lighter oils such as sweet almond, apricot kernel, peach kernel, grapeseed, safflower, sunflower or soya oil are the most suitable for massage and can be used 100%. Thicker, richer oils such as jojoba, avocado pear and wheatgerm are too heavy and sticky to be used on their own, although they may be added in small quantities to improve the absorption and nourish skin. You may wish to avoid carrier oils with a strong smell such as sesame and walnut.

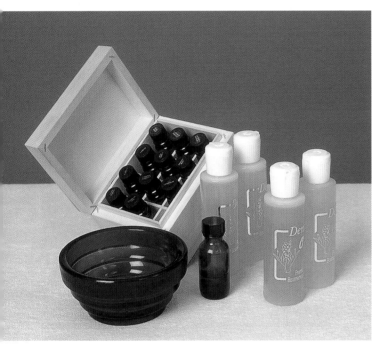

Carrier oils are necessary for blending with your essential oils, so that your hands can move smoothly over your lover's body.

Sweet almond oil is probably the most popular carrier oil.

Following is a brief outline of some of the most commonly used carrier oils. These can be used 100% as a base oil.

SWEET ALMOND OIL

Probably the most widely used carrier oil — favored by Napoleon's wife Josephine and the beauty industry. Highly recommended as it is easily absorbed, does not have a strong odour and is not thick or heavy.
Contains: rich in vitamins including vitamin E and fatty acids.
Uses: all skin types, especially dry, sensitive, inflamed or prematurely aged skin. Good for itchy skin conditions.

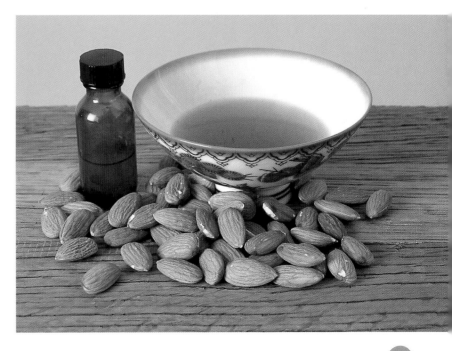

APRICOT KERNEL OIL

A pale, yellowish oil similar to sweet almond oil although more expensive as less is produced.

Contains: vitamins, minerals and fatty acids.

Uses: all skin types, especially dry or sensitive. Ideal as a facial oil or as a natural moisturiser as it helps to feed and regenerate the skin.

The following to be added, if desired, in small quantities (approximately 10%):

JOJOBA

A thick, highly penetrating yellow oil widely used by the cosmetics industry in both skin and hair preparations. Expensive, but worth it.

Contains: proteins, minerals, vitamins and a waxy substance that mimics collagen.

Uses: all skin types — eczema, psoriasis and skin conditions.

AVOCADO PEAR

A dark, rich, green colour — if it is yellow it has been refined so do not buy it. It is very viscous and penetrating.

Contains: vitamins A, B and D, lecithin, fatty acids.

Uses: very nourishing. Ideal for dry, dehydrated and mature skin.

WHEATGERM

A rich, orange brown oil, very nourishing but has a strong odour.

Contains: vitamin E, proteins, minerals.

Uses: added as it is anti-oxidant and a preservative prolonging the life of a blend. Helps dry, cracked skin, mature skin, eczema, psoriasis. Prevents stretch marks and premature ageing.

Adding essential oils to your carrier oil is an excellent way to enhance your treatment.

The vitamin E contained in Wheatgerm Oil makes it particularly suitable for soothing dry or irritated skin.

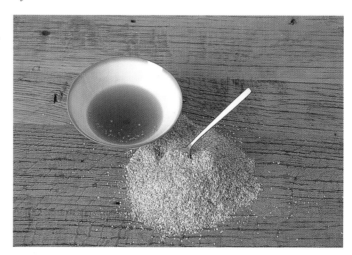

Make sure Avocado Oil is dark green – do not buy it if it is yellow.

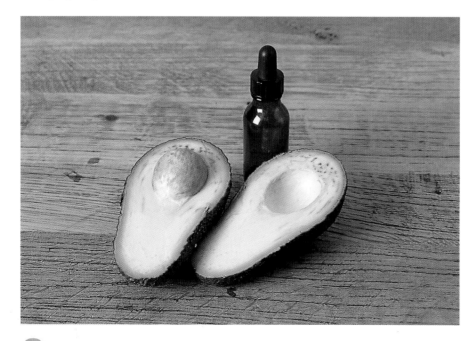

CHECKLIST

What You Need For Sensual Massage:
- Peace and quiet
- A well-heated room
- Dim lights/candlelight
- A thick duvet, sleeping bag, blankets or futon to create a firm, well-padded surface
- Oil burner-if you have one
- A selection of towels
- Pillows and cushions
- Carrier oil/essential oils
- Small bowl or a flip top bottle

Essential Oils

Essential oils can greatly enhance a sensual massage and increase sexual arousal. The combination of touch and aroma is very potent. However it is vital to remember that pure essential oils are highly concentrated and should NEVER be applied undiluted. They should be blended with a suitable carrier oil in the appropriate dilution. Please follow these guidelines:

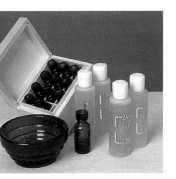

- 3 drops of essential oil to 10 mls of carrier oil
- 4-5 drops to 15 mls of carrier oil
- 6 drops to 20 mls of carrier oil

A teaspoon holds approximately 5 mls and a complete sensual massage should never require more than 4 teaspoons of carrier oil (i.e. 20 mls). Do not be tempted to use more essential oil. This will not make the formulation more effective and it could create an unpleasant side effect such as a skin reaction.

To begin with, choose just ONE of the 15 essential oils outlined. After you have mixed up your love potion, rub a small amount onto your lover's hand and smell it. If the aroma is pleasurable to BOTH of you then use it — if you both like the aroma it will have the desired effect. No one particular essential oil will appeal to everyone — aroma preference is a matter of personal taste. After you have acquired several essential oils try blending two or three together to create your own special recipes.

OTHER WAYS OF USING EROTIC OILS

There are numerous ways of using essential oils. Some of the simplest and most effective techniques for you and your lover are outlined here.

BATH — fill the bath and sprinkle in SIX drops of your chosen undiluted oil. Disperse the oil thoroughly and close the door so that the precious vapours cannot escape. Soak in the bath and allow the aromas to envelop you. Why not surround the bath with flickering candles and ask your lover to join you?

SITZ baths and BIDETS —Sitz baths are highly beneficial in cases of cystitis, vaginal discharges, thrush etc. They are also invaluable for protecting against infections and viruses. Simply add six drops of essential oil to a bidet or a bowl of hand-hot water. Agitate thoroughly and sit in it for about ten minutes.

SCENTING — scenting the room with essential oils helps to create the perfect sensual environment.

The oils shown in the following directory are listed in alphabetical order by Latin name.

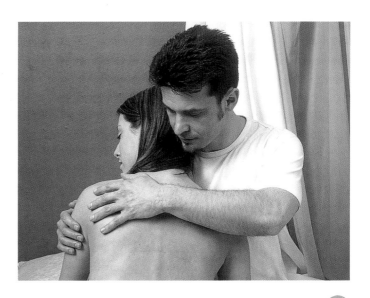

The combination of touch and aroma is irresistible, and enhances your sensual pleasure.

FRANKINCENSE

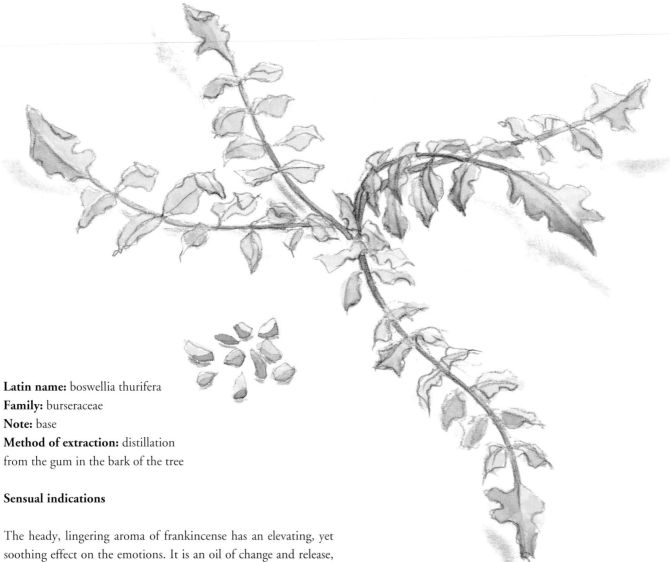

Latin name: boswellia thurifera
Family: burseraceae
Note: base
Method of extraction: distillation
from the gum in the bark of the tree

Sensual indications

The heady, lingering aroma of frankincense has an elevating, yet soothing effect on the emotions. It is an oil of change and release, which allows past traumas and anxieties to gently melt away. Sometimes, even when a relationship has finished, one or both lovers can cling to the memories and harbor feelings of deep sadness, regret, guilt or failure. It is vital to cut the ties from one relationship before embarking on a new one if you are to succeed. Difficulties experienced with one lover, if left unresolved, will re-emerge and create problems. Frankincense is the oil of enlightenment, which enables these deep-seated emotions to rise to the surface and fade away.

Frankincense is a deep and mysterious essential oil favored by the Egyptians thousands of years ago. It is ideal for re-kindling the passion in a stale relationship. With the aid of frankincense there is no reason why any loving couple should get bored.

Other uses

- Urinary infections, cystitis, thrush, painful menstruation, scanty and heavy menstruation.
- Excellent for skin care as its rejuvenating properties prevent aging, revitalize mature skin and may help wrinkles. Add a few drops to your moisturizer or to a jar of pure organic skin cream.

Contra-indications

None.

YLANG YLANG

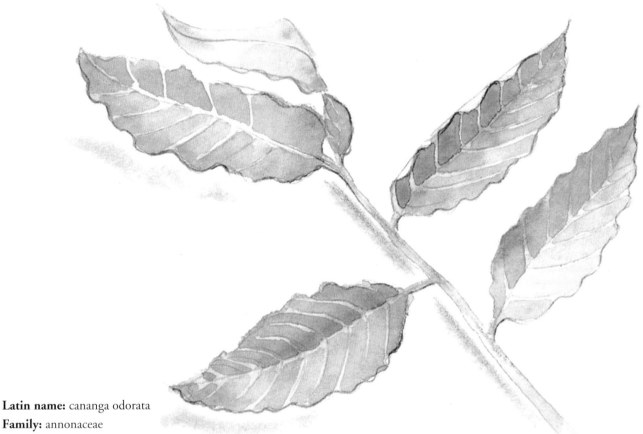

Latin name: cananga odorata
Family: annonaceae
Note: base
Method of extraction: distillation
from the freshly picked flowers

Sensual indications

Ylang ylang is renowned for its aphrodisiac properties and in Indonesia the flowers are spread on the beds of newlyweds. It dispels any apprehension the couple may have and creates a sense of euphoria.

This oil is deeply relaxing and is excellent for releasing anxiety and tension. Anger, which has welled up because of the frustrations of the day, can be rapidly inhibited and released.

States of fear can be soothed by sensual massage with essential oil of ylang ylang. For women who have fear of intimacy either because they are inexperienced or because of former traumas this oil is invaluable. It gently melts away the fear, giving rise to a sense of deep relaxation.

The aroma is exceedingly exotic, sweet and erotic, and ylang ylang is used extensively in high-class perfumery. If you use ylang ylang in your sensual massage oil why not make double the quantity and use it as a perfume oil afterwards to attract your lover?

Other uses

Skin — all skin care, particularly oily skin. Ylang ylang also encourages hair growth — a few drops in your final rinse will leave a lingering sensual aroma.

Contra-indications

Take care not to exceed the recommended dose or the heady aroma of ylang ylang may cause a headache.

CEDARWOOD

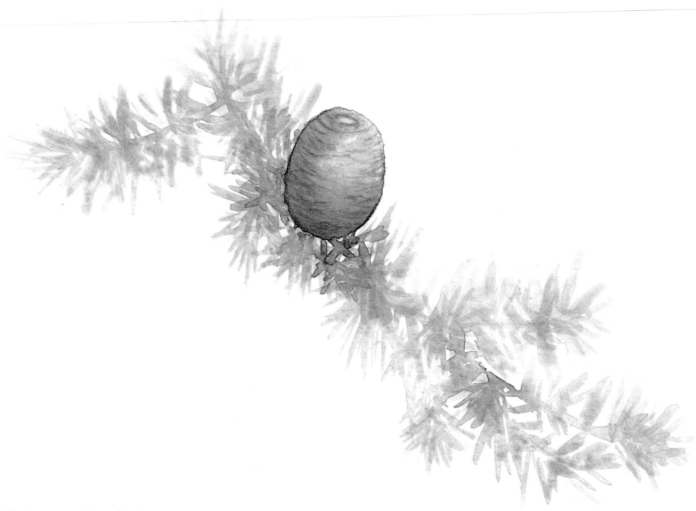

Latin name: cedrus atlantica
Family: pinaceae
Note: base
Method of extraction: distillation from wood

Sensual indications

The deliciously woody aroma of this essential oil will enable you and your lover to slowly unwind after a stressful day. This calming and soothing oil is beneficial for all states of tension and helps to melt away all anger and frustration.

Cedarwood is a popular choice for both men and women and is particularly useful for prolonging foreplay. It is a sedative oil, which helps to calm down the mind and will allow you both to experience total relaxation, contentment and satisfaction.

Other uses

Recommended for the urinary tract, alleviating burning sensations and itching which can occur with vaginal infections and discharges. Sprinkle 4-5 drops of cedarwood into a bowl of warm water or a bidet and sit in it for approximately 10 minutes to gain maximum benefit.

Contra-indications

- Best avoided during pregnancy.
- Avoid Texas cedarwood and Virginian cedarwood which can cause skin sensitization.

NEROLI (ORANGE BLOSSOM)

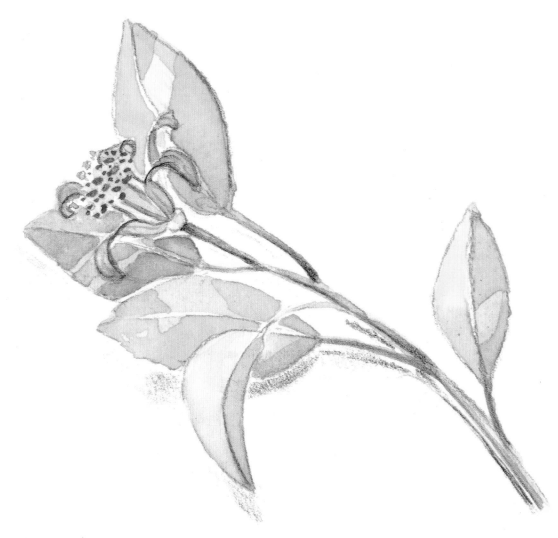

Latin name: citrus aurantium var. amara
Family: rutaceae
Note: base
Method of extraction: distillation from the flowers

Sensual indications

The delicious, sweet and floral fragrance of this oil makes it a popular (although expensive) choice as an aphrodisiac. Orange flowers have traditionally been used in bridal bouquets to allay any nervous apprehension prior to the honeymoon night. Neroli oil is used extensively in high-class perfumery as it has the most exquisite aroma.

This oil is one of the most effective remedies for emotional problems and can be used for any stress-related disorder. It can even counteract panic attacks. If a lover is very fearful or has an aversion to any bodily contact or sexual advances, neroli is the perfect choice. If abuse has taken place then the terror can lead to frigidity and negative emotions such as guilt. Neroli can help soothe and heal the emotional scarring which remains, and instil a feeling of euphoria and confidence.

Other uses

Skin care — all types of skin especially sensitive and mature. Neroli is rejuvenating and works wonders for wrinkles. It can also help to prevent stretch marks and reduces scars.

Contra-indications

None.

BERGAMOT

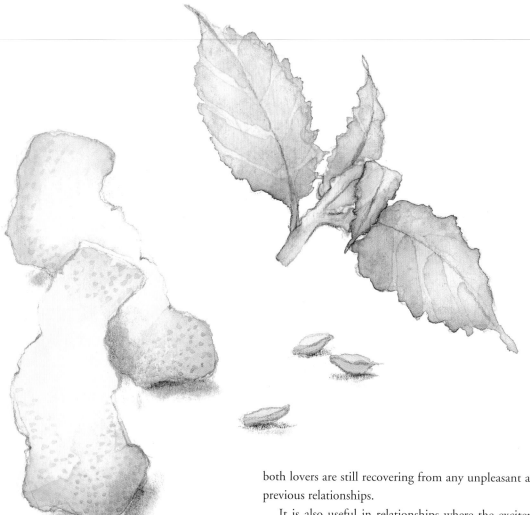

Latin name: citrus bergamia
Family: rutaceae
Note: base
Method of extraction: expression from the peel of the fruit

Sensual indications

Bergamot has a wonderfully refreshing, sweet citrus aroma. It has a potent effect on the emotions — uplifting the mind and alleviating states of depression and negativity. It will help to inspire confidence and stimulates those with a low sexual appetite.

Bergamot has the ability to open up the heart and to heal old wounds, and is ideal for use in new relationships where one or both lovers are still recovering from any unpleasant after-effects of previous relationships.

It is also useful in relationships where the excitement of love-making has dwindled. It helps to add a new sparkle to your love life.

Other uses

Bergamot has a strong affinity for the genito-urinary system and is invaluable for relieving as well as preventing cystitis, vaginal discharges and sexually transmitted diseases such as herpes. Add 4-6 drops to a bowl of warm water or to the bidet, thoroughly mix and sit in the bowl for approximately 10 minutes. Repeat this procedure at least twice today until the infection resolves.

Contra-indications

Do not apply bergamot prior to sun bathing as it increases the photosensitivity of the skin.

JASMINE

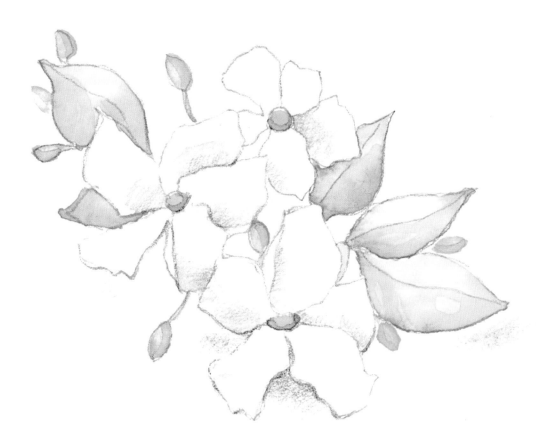

Latin name: jasminum officinale
Family: oleaceae
Note: base
Method of extraction: solvent extraction from the flowers

Sensual indications

Jasmine is often referred to as the 'King of essential oils'. It brings out the seducer or the seductress in you. A jasmine woman is alluring, radiating confidence and vibrancy, and is irresistible to a man. It helps to bring out all those hidden sexual desires and is one of the most renowned aphrodisiacs.

The exquisite, exotic, heady aroma is wonderful for inducing optimism, confidence and euphoria. Although it is very expensive it is well worth the investment. Indulge yourself and release your inhibitions!

Where there is a loss of libido, jasmine can alleviate frigidity and impotence. It also helps to strengthen the male sex organs and is therefore useful for problems such as premature ejaculation.

Jasmine is excellent for infertility problems. Not only does it relieve the stress and anxiety (surrounding the longing for a baby) but also increases the production of semen.

Other uses

- Childbirth — jasmine relieves the pain, promotes the birth, prevents postnatal depression and encourages a good milk supply.
- Reduces stretch marks and scars.

Contra-indications

None.

MYRTLE

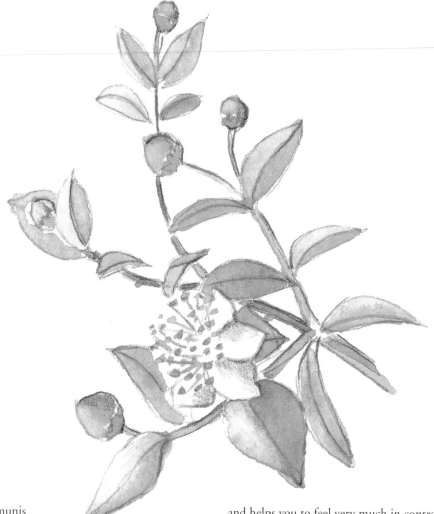

Latin name: myrtus communis
Family: myrtaceae
Note: middle
Method of extraction: distillation from the leaves, twigs and flowers

Sensual indications

In Greek mythology Aphrodite, the goddess of love, chose sprigs of myrtle in order to hide her naked body, and it is fascinating that the myrtle plant has leaves shaped like a vagina. Centuries ago the Kama Sutra suggested that myrtle could be used to evoke sexual desire. It appears that myrtle enables a woman to contact her Aphrodite goddess energy within — her loving sensual energy.

Put six drops into your bath to induce not only sexual desire but also a sense of calmness. Myrtle relieves anger and frustration and helps you to feel very much in control of the your own sexuality. This inspiring essential oil enables a woman to know what she wants and gives her the ability to express her sexual desires.

Myrtle is an excellent oil for boosting the immune system and can offer additional protection against sexual diseases.

Other uses

- Skin care — in the sixteenth century myrtle was a major ingredient of 'Angel Water', used in a lotion as a tonic and astringent.
- Colds, coughs and flu as a chest and back rub.

Contra-indications

None.

GERANIUM

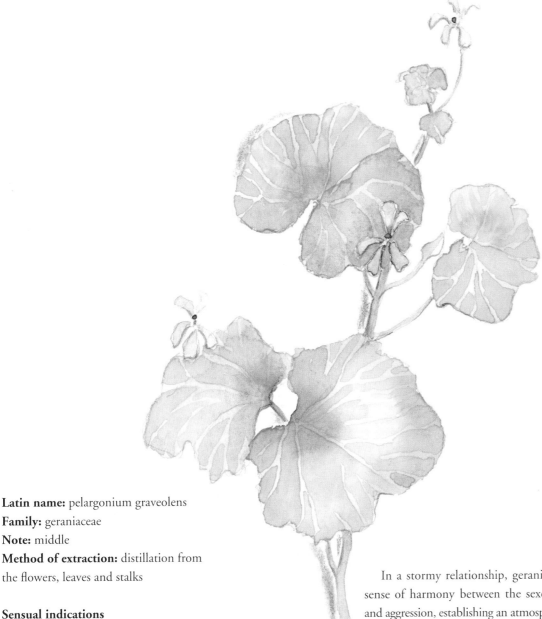

Latin name: pelargonium graveolens
Family: geraniaceae
Note: middle
Method of extraction: distillation from
the flowers, leaves and stalks

Sensual indications

The balancing properties of geranium are particularly beneficial for women, who are very fond of this essential oil. It is a superb oil for all female problems particularly PMS and infertility and also for dispelling anxiety and apprehension.

It may be useful at the beginning of a relationship when one or both lovers are nervous about what lies ahead of them. If either of them have recently broken up with their lover, or feel dejected then the healing properties of geranium will help to soothe past wounds and boost morale.

In a stormy relationship, geranium is excellent for creating a sense of harmony between the sexes. It quells anger, frustration and aggression, establishing an atmosphere of peace and contentment.

Other uses

* Varicose veins.
* Excellent for all types of skin whether oily, dry or combination. Add a few drops to your moisturizing cream.

Contra-indications

None.

BLACK PEPPER

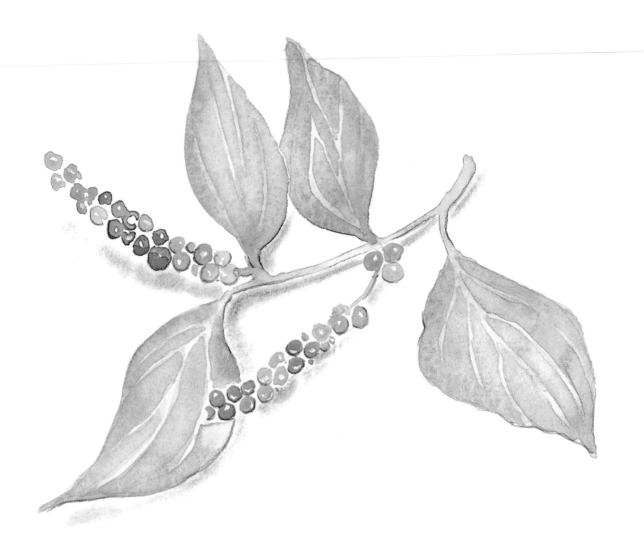

Latin name: piper nigrum

Family: piperaceae

Note: middle

Method of extraction: distillation from the peppercorns, dried and crushed

Sensual indications

The spicy, hot and pungent aroma of black pepper is ideal for awakening and increasing sexual desire. It is one of the most effective essential oils for alleviating impotency and boosting male sexual energy. Impotency is a problem for the majority of men at some stage in their lives and may be due to tension, physical, or emotional exhaustion or a lack of confidence. The peppery aroma will stimulate both body and mind into action. Black pepper has the ability to give strength and stamina and therefore can be useful in cases of premature ejaculation.

Other uses

- Poor circulation
- All muscular aches and pains
- Digestive disorders such as constipation — massage the abdomen in a clockwise direction when necessary.

Contra-indications

None.

PATCHOULI

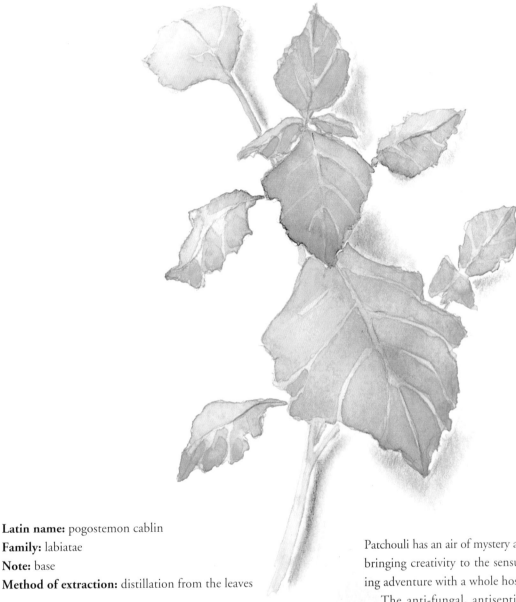

Latin name: pogostemon cablin
Family: labiatae
Note: base
Method of extraction: distillation from the leaves

Sensual indications

Patchouli was an extremely popular oil in the 1960s, favored by the 'hippies' who advocated love and peace. Most people will either love or hate its earthly, musty, heavy aroma. Like a good wine it definitely improves with age.

This oil is renowned for its success in treating impotence and especially frigidity, although check out the aroma first — if you dislike the smell then it will obviously not turn you on. Patchouli is particularly suitable for women with a low sexual response and can help those who have never experienced an orgasm.

Patchouli has an air of mystery and can help couples stuck in a rut by bringing creativity to the sensual relationship. Sex is a never-ending adventure with a whole host of new experiences before you.

The anti-fungal, antiseptic properties of patchouli make it ideal for vaginal infections and thrush. Put 4-6 drops in a bidet or a bowl of warm water and soak for ten minutes.

Other uses

Skin care — especially dry, cracked, chapped skin, fungal infections, allergies such as eczema, mature skin.

Contra-indications

None.

ROSEWOOD

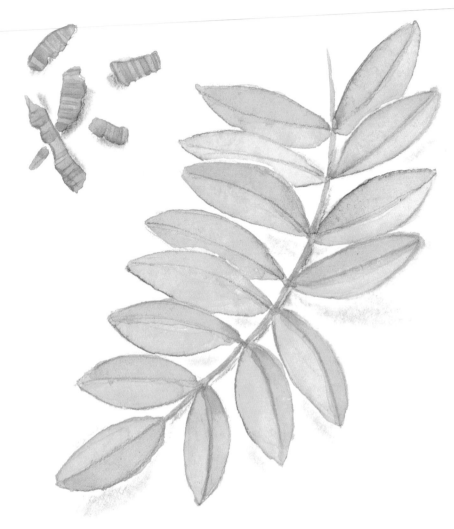

Latin name: aniba rosaeodora
Family: lauraceae
Note: middle
Method of Extraction: Distillation of the wood chippings

Sensual indications

The sweet, woody, floral aroma of rosewood can bring peace and tranquillity to a troubled mind. It is marvellous as an antidepressant, uplifting both body and mind and dispelling lethargy and exhaustion. A sensual massage at the end of a stressful day with essential oil of rosewood is the perfect way to unwind and to get into the right mood for a night of passion.

Rosewood is a remarkable aphrodisiac, helping to combat both frigidity and impotence. The spicy hint in this aroma can inject new life into a dwindling relationship, re-kindling sensual feelings.

This essential oil is also invaluable for dispelling emotional blockages created by a previous relationship they may put up barriers to protect against future trauma.

Other uses

*   Boosts the immune system
*   All skin care. Rosewood rejuvenates the skin. Add a few drops to your moisturizer to prevent aging and banish wrinkles.

Contra-indications

None.

ROSE

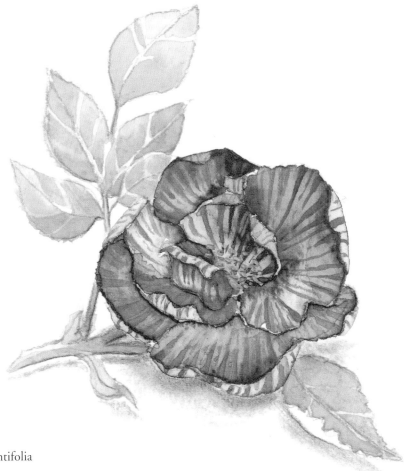

Latin name: rosa damascena/centifolia
Family: rosaceae
Note: base
Method of extraction: distillation from the fresh petals

Sensual indications

Rose is often referred to as the 'Queen of Essential Oils' and is traditionally associated with Venus, the goddess of love and beauty. This oil, unfortunately mostly in a synthetic form is found in almost all women's perfumes and in almost 50% of men's fragrances. Its reputation as an aphrodisiac is second to none.

The deep, rich and sweet floral scent of rose oil will captivate any woman. Although expensive, it is well worth the investment. It is common practice to send a dozen roses to express love but a small bottle of essential oil of rose will last longer, and will bring even more pleasure. Always be suspicious of cheap rose oil, which is synthetic and will not work.

Rose has a profound effect on the emotions, alleviating bitterness and resentment. It can therefore be useful to release any unresolved feelings lingering from past relationships. It makes a woman feel very feminine and positive about herself and thus is useful where there is low esteem or feelings of uncleanness, which can emerge after rape. Rose is the most effective oil for infertility. It prepares the womb for conception and in the male increases the production of semen.

Other uses

- Skin — all skin types especially dry, mature, sensitive and thread veins.
- All female problems — menopause, PMS, heavy or scanty menstruation.

Contra-indications

None.

CLARY SAGE

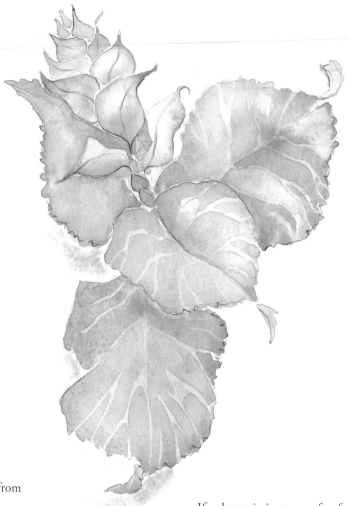

Latin name: salvia sclarea
Family: labiatae
Note: middle
Method of extraction: distillation from
the flowering tops and leaves

Sensual indications

Clary sage is a renowned aphrodisiac capable of increasing libido in both men and women. The intoxicating heady, sweet aroma of this oil has a sedative yet euphoric effect on the mind, dispelling general debility whether it is physical, mental, nervous or sexual. A relaxed nervous system will always respond much more readily than an over-anxious system. Clary sage is useful for erection difficulties particularly when they are related to anxiety and tension.

Clary sage instils a sense of well-being and optimism and is invaluable when life is particularly difficult. It provides an alternative to tranquillisers and one or two drops can be sprinkled onto a tissue and inhaled as an alternative to drugs such as Valium or Prozac.

If a lover is insecure, fearful or even panicky and puts up blocks to any sexual advances, clary sage is an excellent oil for breaking down the barriers.

Clary sage is also effective for increasing both male and female infertility.

Other uses

- Pre-menstrual syndrome (PMS), painful and scanty menstruation.
- Clary sage is a tonic for the womb and helps to balance the hormones.

Contra-indications

Do not take alcohol and clary sage together as this can lead to headaches and nightmares and exaggerate the effects of alcohol.

SANDALWOOD

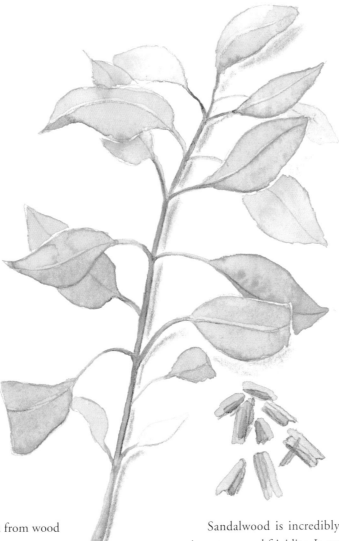

Latin name: santalum album
Family: santalaceae
Note: base
Method of extraction: distillation from wood

Sensual indications

Sandalwood has been used for thousands of years all over the East. In India it is used in ayurvedic medicine and is combined with rose to make the perfume 'aytar'. Both men and women find the soft, sweet woody aroma of sandalwood oil irresistible, which makes it an ideal choice for sensual massage.

This essential oil is deeply relaxing and is renowned for its ability to gently soothe away tension. As you massage with sandalwood it seems to fill the body with a warm glow and a sense of deep satisfaction and contentment. It is a sedative and peaceful oil and is invaluable for promoting harmony within a stormy relationship. Try it after a disagreement and notice how calm and mellow you become.

Sandalwood is incredibly seductive and is helpful for both impotence and frigidity. It can increase the initial response and lift your sex life to new heights. You will both feel so relaxed that it will prolong your lovemaking and counteract premature ejaculation. Sandalwood is one of the best oils to use for genito-urinary infections and 4-6 drops can be used in a sitz bath or bowl of warm water daily to prevent infections from occurring.

Other uses

Skin — particularly good for dry or cracked skin. It can be blended with carrier oil to make an excellent after-shave.

Contra-indications

None.

GINGER

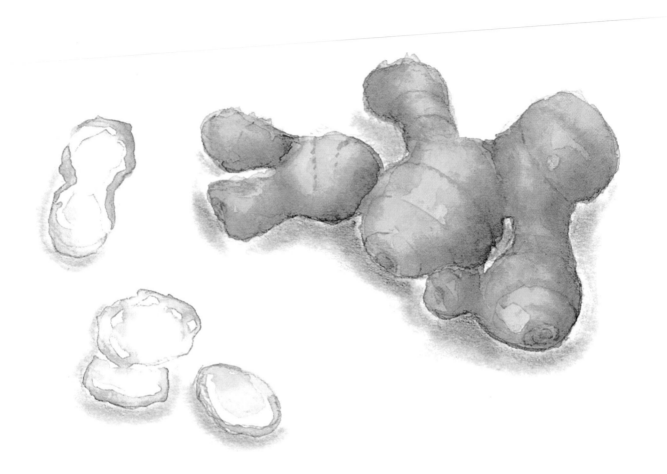

Latin name: zingiber officinale
Family: zingiberaceae
Note: top
Method of extraction: distillation from the unpeeled, dried ground root.

Sensual indications

This is certainly the oil to spice up your love life. If you feel bored or stuck in a rut then the hot, zingy aroma of ginger will add a whole new dimension to your relationship.

Ginger is one of the best oils for male impotence and a weak erection. Often the appetite may be normal with a strong desire to make love but the ability is not there. Where there is no sexual response, or arousal is very slow and laboured, ginger is highly recommended. The fiery, warming properties can help to counteract not only physical inability but also sexual coldness and disinterest.

Ginger will fill a man with courage and is therefore indicated for a male who in a previous relationship may have had his confidence shattered by a lover who told him he was 'not good enough'.

In a new relationship it is usual to feel somewhat nervous with 'butterflies in the stomach'. Ginger is a classic remedy for nausea and will help to settle the digestive system and the nerves and restore confidence.

Other uses

* Poor circulation
* Muscular aches and pains where pain relief is required, coldness and stiffness in the joints.

Contra-indications

None.

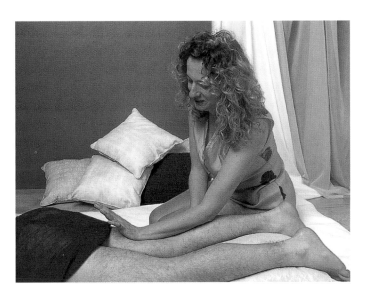

Once you are comfortable with the basic massage techniques, enjoy experimenting to create your own strokes.

There are many different massage techniques. The magic of massage is that it is simple and intuitive. These basic techniques will enable you to perform a complete sensual massage. Once you have mastered these movements you will find yourself inventing your own strokes.

APPLYING THE OIL

Oil should NEVER be poured directly onto the body. This would be a shock to the system especially if the oil is cold. If possible warm your oil beforehand by putting it on top of a radiator, in front of a heater or standing it in a bowl of hot water. The oil may be kept either in a flip-top bottle or you may dispense a small amount into a small bowl or saucer but be careful not to knock it over.

Warm cold hands before you start by rubbing them together vigorously or immersing them in hot water for a few minutes. Now pour a small quantity (about half a teaspoon) into the palm of one hand. Rub your hands together to warm the oil slightly before applying it. Lower your hands gently and begin to apply the oil using one of the stroking movements described in this chapter.

Once you have made contact with your lover, do not break it or you will destroy the continuity of your massage. Ideally your massage should feel like one continuous flow of movements. If you require more oil, then ensure that you keep one hand in contact with the body.

A very common error is to use too much carrier oil which can make the receiver feel uncomfortable and sticky and can stain their clothes. It is also nearly impossible to perform some of the basic techniques with too much oil.

Before you master the techniques of massage, here are a few basic guidelines to help you.

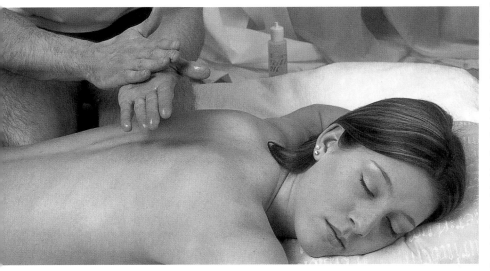

Cold hands and oil can spoil your lover's mood, so always warm oil in your hands before applying.

MASSAGE TIPS

- Center yourself prior to the massage so that you are totally relaxed. Never give a massage when you are angry, anxious or depleted.
- Always wash and warm your hands before you start.
- Check that fingernails are short and clean.
- Remove all jewelry to avoid scratching.
- Try to make your massage feel like one continuous movement.
- Mold your hands to the contours of the body.
- When giving a massage, ask your lover to let you know if he/she is particularly enjoying a certain movement or if they find a movement uncomfortable. Massage should always be pleasurable. Keep talking to a minimum.
- Experiment with different pressures — vary it from light to strong according to which pressure your lover likes. Never put heavy pressure on the bony areas.
- Try different rhythms — slow and steady or firm and brisk.
- Work with your eyes closed to heighten and increase your sensitivity.
- Once you have made contact with your lover try not to break it. If you need to collect more oil or move from one part of the body to the next try to maintain one hand in contact.
- As you massage, be aware of your own posture so that you do not strain or hurt yourself. Make sure that your shoulders are relaxed so that the healing energy can flow freely through your hands.

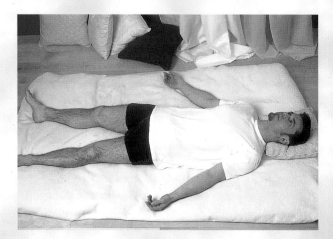

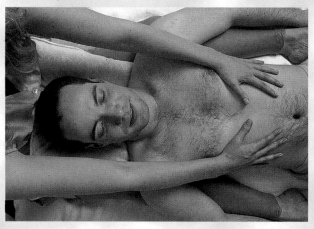

Remember to center yourself before beginning a massage, so that your are relaxed and free of tension.

Experiment with different techniques and positions to find those that suit both yourself and your lover.

STROKING

Stroking forms the basis of a sensual massage. In fact by varying your stroking movements you could carry out a complete sensual massage as it can be performed on any area of the body and can be varied enormously by changing the speed or pressure of the strokes.

Your movements can be long or short, firm or gentle, slow or brisk. These variations will help to keep your lover's interest and he/she will wonder what is coming next.

Stroking signals the beginning and the end of a sensual massage and allows you to flow from one technique to the next. It is a deeply relaxing movement, which establishes a sense of trust and allows your lover to feel loving and yielding as you gently caress the body. Stress and tension is relieved as muscles relax, circulation improves and toxins are eliminated from the body.

To perform this technique, the palms of both hands are used as you glide over the surface of the skin molding your hands to the contours of the body part on which you are working. A steady, even pressure is applied through the palms of your hands as you glide over the body. On the return stroke use a feather light touch to return to your starting point. There are many different stroking techniques. Once you have mastered these it is a natural next step to create your own special strokes. Always use your intuition and be spontaneous.

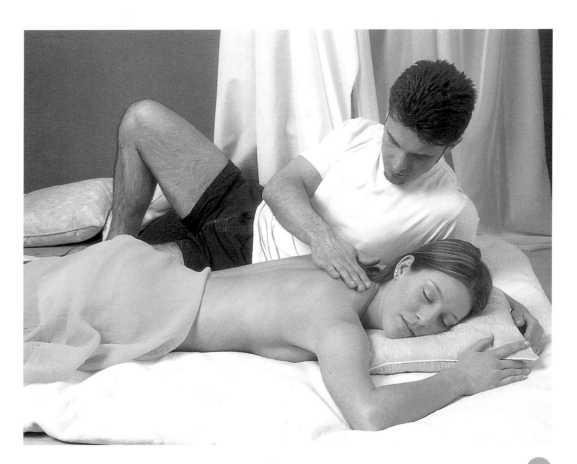

Stroking is one of the most important elements of a sensual massage. You will feel your lover relax as tension melts away.

LONG STROKING

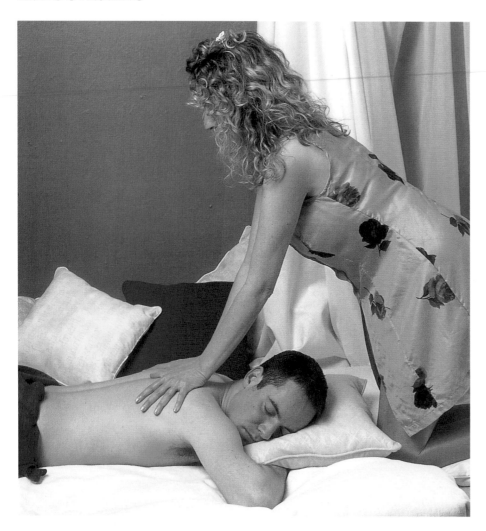

To perform this movement, position yourself in a comfortable kneeling position at your lover's head. Place the palms of your relaxed hands side by side on their shoulders.

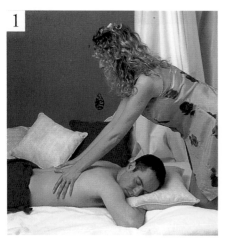
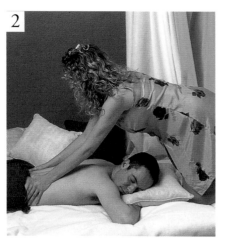

1.Stroke the entire back, using the palms of both hands, gliding down both sides of the spine.

2. When you reach the base of the spine, separate your hands and glide over the buttocks.

Allow your hands to glide back to your starting point without any pressure. Notice your lover's breathing as you perform this movement as well as your own. You will find that your breathing starts to follow the same pattern. You and your lover start to breath in and out at the same pace. A strong, deeply intimate connection is established.

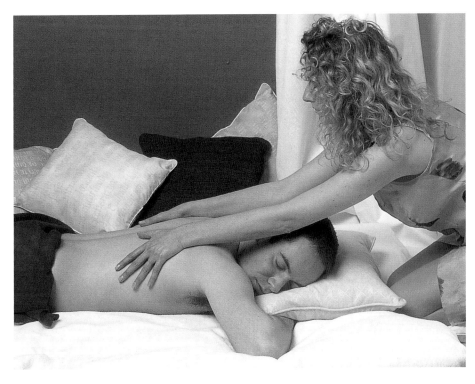

CIRCLE STROKING
(ONE HAND FOLLOWING THE OTHER)

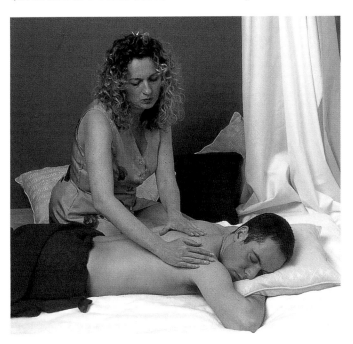

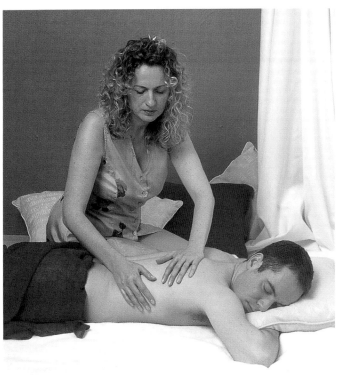

Position yourself to one side of your lover and place both hands on one side of the body around the shoulder blade. Using the whole of the palms of your hands, make large stroking movements in a circular motion.

Your hands will cross over as you perform your circles. Although you will have to lift one hand over the other, always keep contact with one hand. You may work right the way down your lover's body towards the buttocks and back up towards the shoulders again.

CIRCLE STROKING
(ONE HAND ON TOP OF THE OTHER)

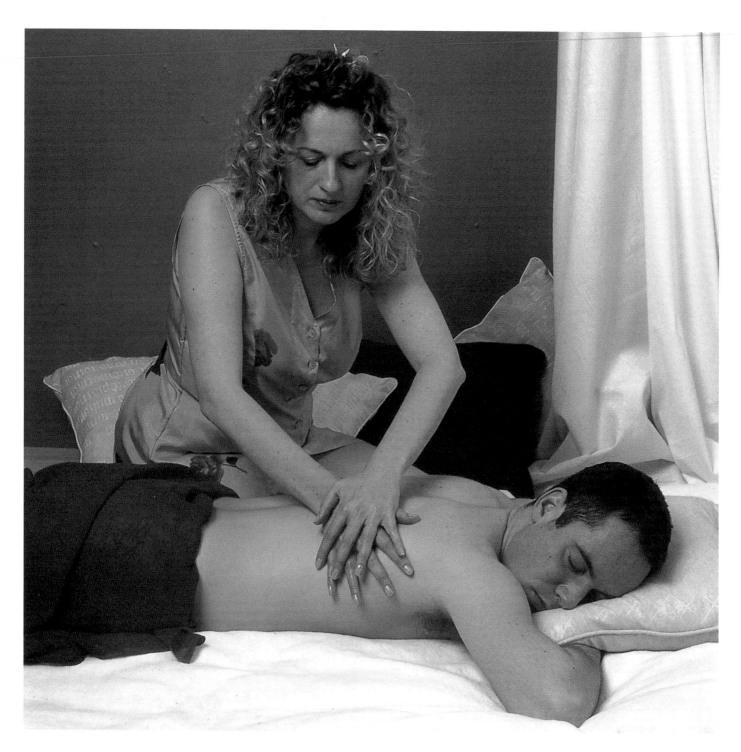

Place one hand flat on top of the other and, using the whole of the hand, make large circular movements working from the top of the shoulder blade down towards the buttocks. Then work from the buttocks up towards the shoulder blade. Repeat on the other side of the spine.

CIRCLE STROKING
(ONE HAND ON TOP OF THE OTHER)

Position yourself at the side of your lover close to the buttocks — or you may even sit astride your lover. Starting at the top of the body, stroke down the back slowly using just the fingertips of one hand so that you are barely touching the skin. One hand follows the other. As your first hand reaches your lover's buttocks, lift it gently off as your other hand commences the movement.

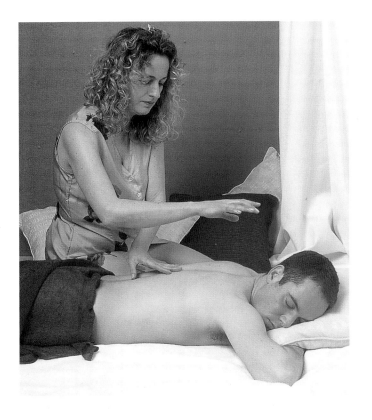

For some of the techniques, you may find sitting astride your lover is more comfortable — as well as making you feel closer.

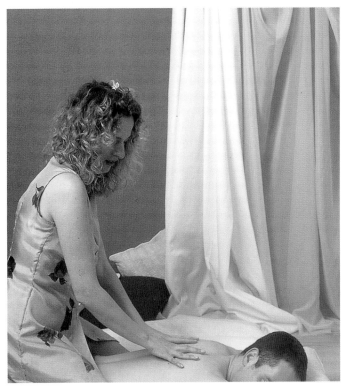

FINGERTIP STROKING – BOTH FINGERTIPS

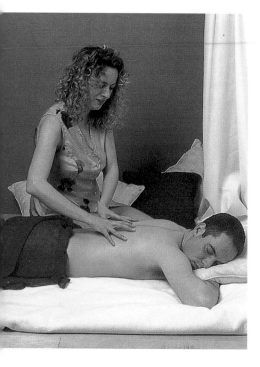

Sitting in the same position gently place both hands, fingertips down, at the top of your lover's shoulders. With both hands, stroke down the body on either side of the spine using just your fingertips. Most people find this movement very erotic.

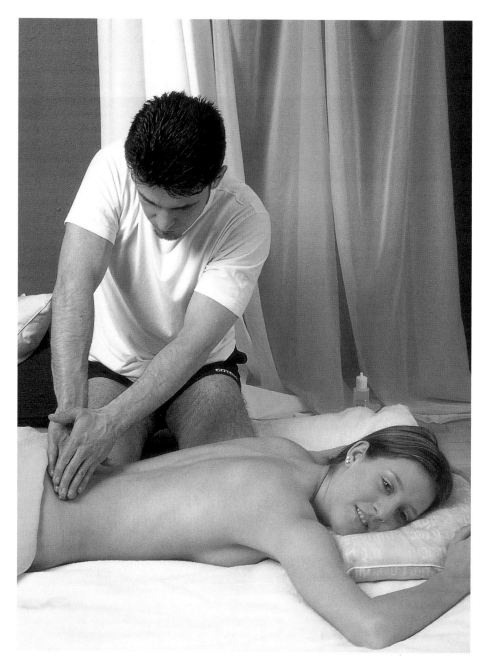

Gentle stroking with both hands is one of the most erotic massage movements.

CAT STROKING

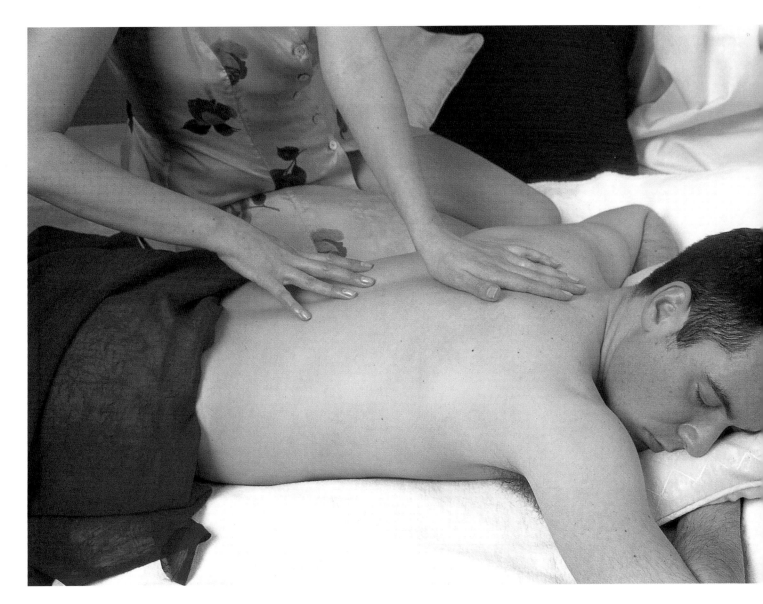

Position yourself to the side of your lover near the buttocks, and place the whole of your right hand palm downward at the base of the neck on the spine. Stroke your hand smoothly down the body using virtually no pressure. As your right hand reaches the buttocks, lift it off and repeat the movement with your left hand. Repeat these movements several times, one hand following the other. It should feel like one continuous movement.

DIAGONAL STROKING

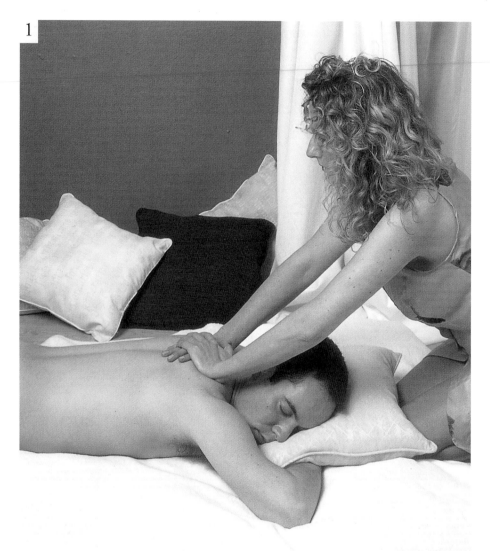

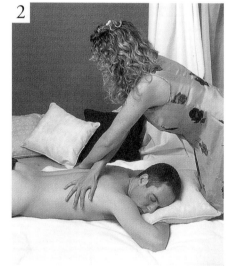

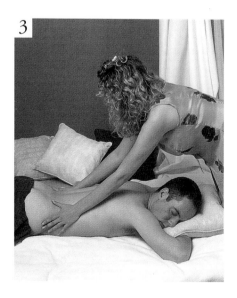

1. Kneel at your lover's head. Allow your hands to float down to rest, one hand crossed on top of the other at the base of the neck.

2. Move them slowly away from each other in opposite directions so that by the time they reach the sides of the body your hands and palms are making a "V".

3. Then slowly glide them back together again. Repeat this movement until you reach the buttocks and then work from the buttocks up to the neck.

STROKING WITH THE BACK OF THE HANDS

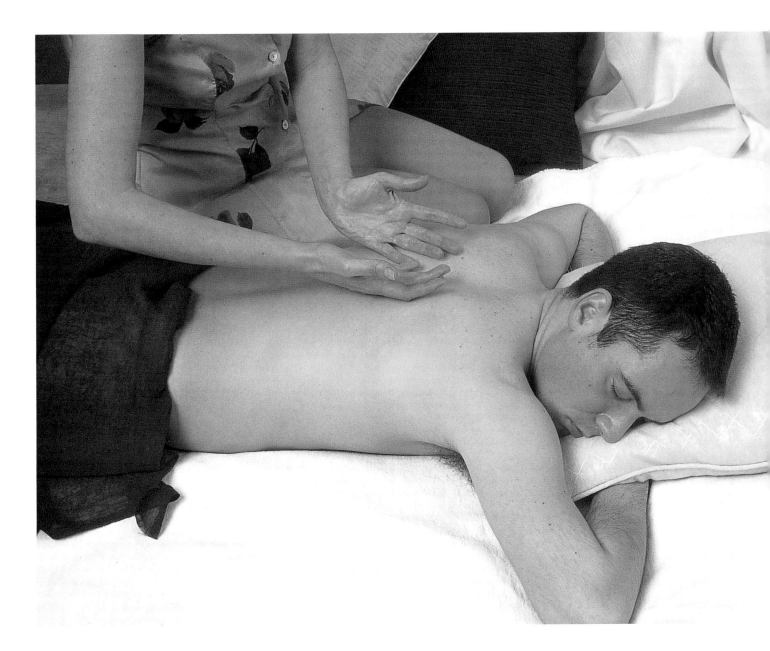

Position yourself to one side of your lover or sit astride him/her. Place the backs of both hands at the top of the body with each hand either side of the spine. Stroke them gently down towards the buttocks. As your hands reach the buttocks, glide back upward to the starting position travelling along the sides of the body.

DEEPER TECHNIQUES

Now that you have relaxed your lover and mastered the flowing movements of stroking you are going to work more deeply into the body with the following techniques.

KNEADING/WRINGING

Kneading is a very beneficial movement. It helps to relax tight muscles, increases the blood supply to the muscles being worked on and helps to get rid of toxins. It is used on fleshy areas such as the thighs, buttocks and hips. Here the shoulder is illustrated. Place your hands flat on the part to be treated and with one hand grasp and squeeze the muscle (not the skin) between your fingers and thumb and bring it towards your other hand. As you release, use the other hand to grasp a new handful of flesh.

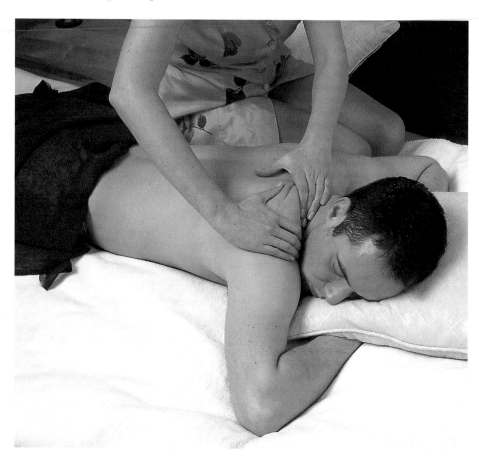

Alternately squeeze and release with both hands as if you are kneading dough. This technique is illustrated on the waist.

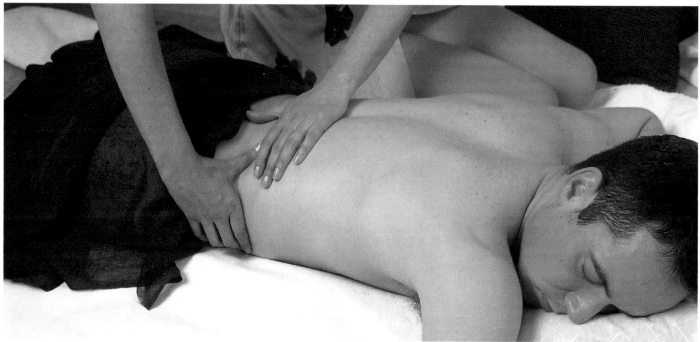

PULLING

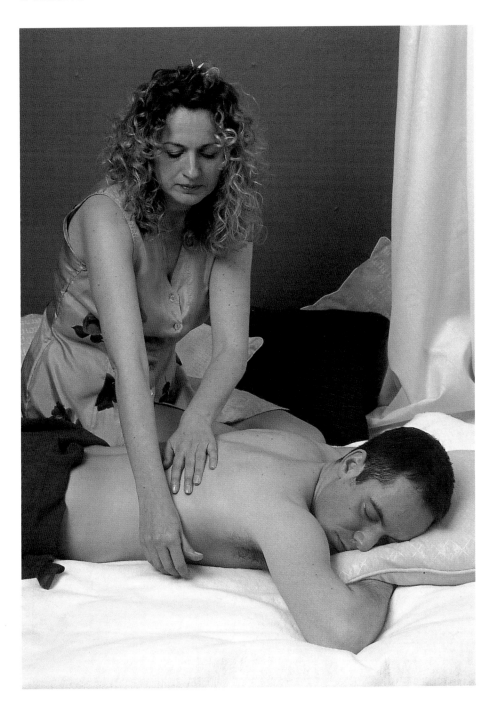

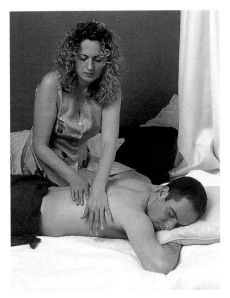

Now pull up the muscle with your other hand. As you pull up with alternate hands, gradually work your way up the side of the back. You may also work down the back. Repeat on the other side of the back.

Kneel comfortably by the side of your lover facing the buttock area. Place both hands on your lover's far side with your fingertips touching the massage surface. Lean over the body and pull up the muscle with your hand.

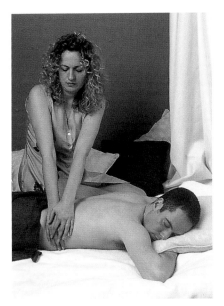

Pulling may also be performed using both hands at the same time.

PUSHING

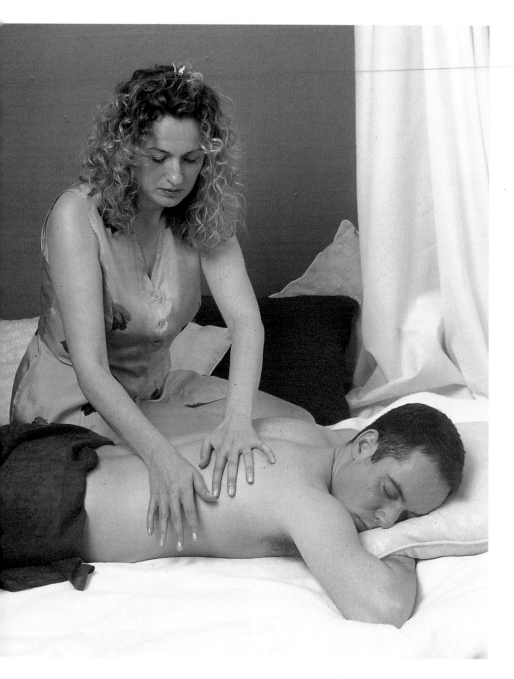

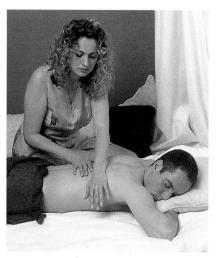

Work your way up your lover's back with pushing movements using alternate hands, one closely following the other. Perform this movement up and down the back. Now try it on the other side.

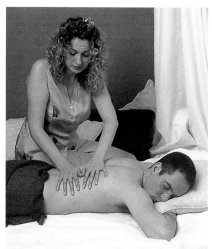

Position yourself as for the pulling technique. Place both hands on the opposite side of the back close to, but NOT touching, the spine itself.

Now try pushing using both hands at the same time.

PRESSURES/FRICTION STROKES

These movements allow you to penetrate deeper into the layers of muscles and to work around joints. Deeper pressure is particularly useful for dispelling tension, which builds up either side of the spine, and around the shoulder blades. Very gentle pressures are also used for the sexual arousal points mentioned in the step-by-step section. The balls of the thumbs are usually used to perform pressure techniques although fingertips, heels of the hands, knuckles or even the elbows may be used.

Remember to always apply pressure gradually and slowly .

never prod sharply into the tissues or dig in with long nails. You will find it easier if you apply just a small amount of oil otherwise your thumbs will slide around and you will only be able to move the skin instead of the deeper tissues underneath.

Use your body weight to add greater depth to your pressure movements-the body is far less delicate than you might think. However, always ask for feedback, as you don't want to inflict any pain and discomfort on your lover.

THUMB PRESSURES

To perform pressure circles on the spinal muscles, position yourself at the side of your lover. Place both hands either side of the spine with the heels of your hands almost touching. Place the balls of your thumbs in the two dimples at the base of the spine. Make small outward circular movements with your thumbs.

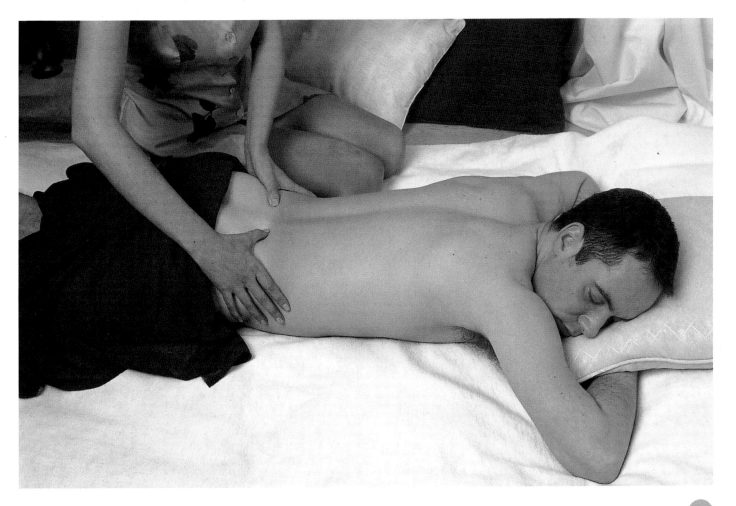

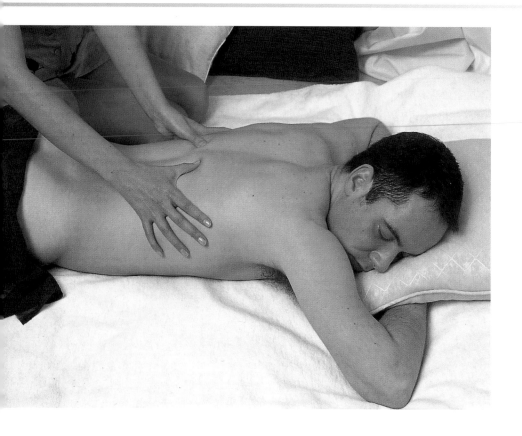

Gradually work up the back until you reach the base of the neck. When you first start it is likely that your thumbs will ache until they become accustomed to the pressure. Make sure that you don't hunch up or you will create knots in your own back and shoulders.

Now try this technique around the shoulder blade. Position yourself close to the shoulder, which you wish to treat. To make it easier you can ask your lover to put their arm behind their back, but if they find it at all uncomfortable or they are asleep leave the arm by their side.

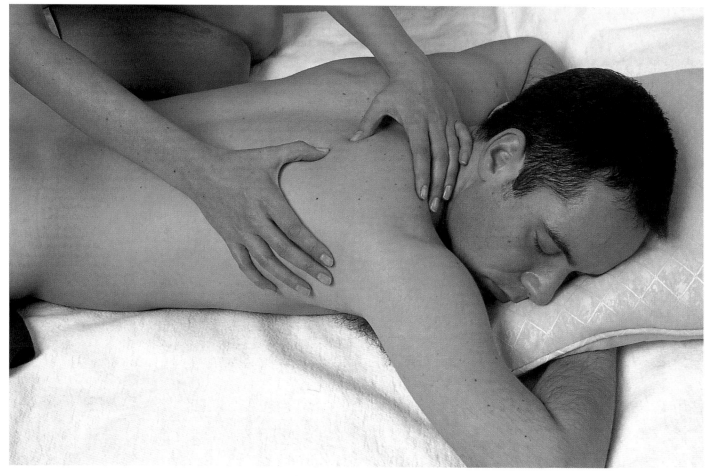

HEEL OF HAND PRESSURE

Instead of using the balls of the thumbs you are now going to use the heels of your hands to apply deep pressure. You will practice this technique on the back of the thigh. This is a wonderful movement for fleshy areas such as the buttocks and thighs.

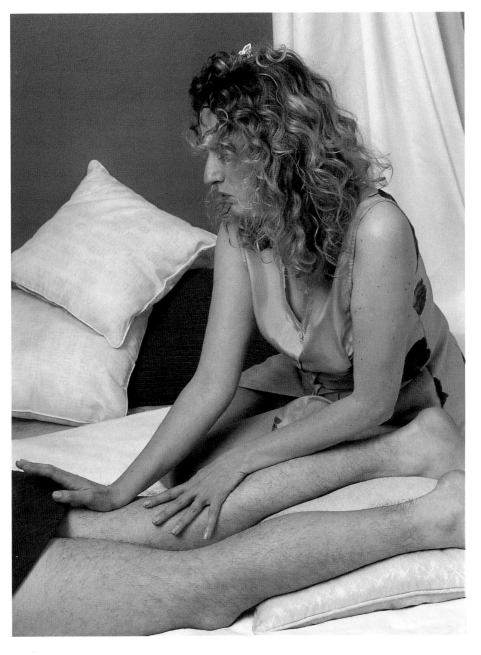

Sit or kneel comfortably at the side of your lover and place the heels of your hands just above the back of the knee. Do NOT press into the back of the knee, which is a very delicate area. Push one hand gently but firmly into the flesh, working up the leg and then push with your other hand. Allow the heels of your hands to move alternately up the back of the thigh.

KNUCKLING

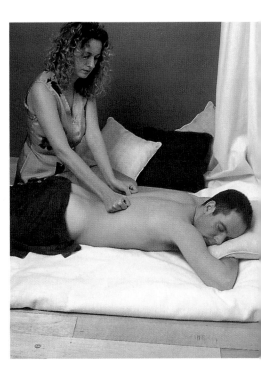

Knuckling feels wonderful when used on the shoulders, back, upper chest, palms of the hands and soles of the feet. Make your hands into loose fists and place them palms down onto the body. Rotate the middle section of your fingers around in a circular direction without taking your hands off the body.

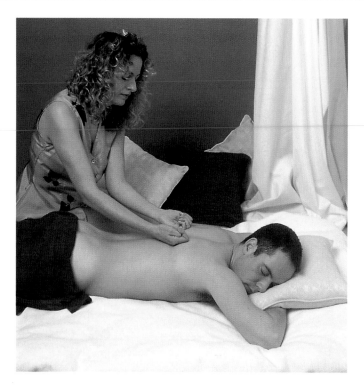

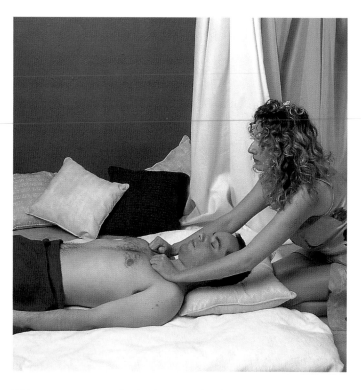

You can also perform this technique using a forward or backward motion instead of a circular motion. Again curl your hands into loose fists, place them on the area to be massaged and slide them forward into the skin. The back is an ideal place to use this technique.

This movement can also be done on the chest area.

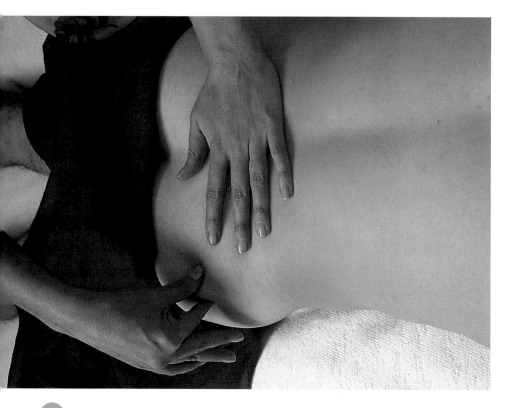

PLUCKING

This technique can be employed over fleshy, muscular areas such as the buttocks and thighs. As well as improving the circulation and toning the skin, plucking is very sensual. Place both hands, palms down, onto the buttocks. Gently pick up small areas of flesh between your thumbs and fingers and let them slip through your hands.

sensual massage
Sequence

This step-by-step guide will enable you to carry out a complete massage on your lover. However, there is no "correct" way to perform a sensual massage — it is important to develop your own style and always use your intuition. You will find that you develop your own techniques and your lover will have his/her special preferences. It is just as good to give a sensual massage as it is to receive one.

You do not need to carry out this complete routine — select your areas and take as much time as you need to complete it. There are NO set rules. Be spontaneous and intuitive. Do not assume that a sensual massage is always intended as a prelude to making love. It is a highly pleasurable experience in its own right, which will bring you closer together and helps to create a harmonious relationship. Remember to set the scene for your sensual massage well in advance.

A full massage would take about one and half hours if you included all the areas of the body. It is far better to concentrate on two or three areas rather than to rush through the whole body. Favorite areas are the back, the head and the feet. Why not try the whole sequence and discover your personal preferences?

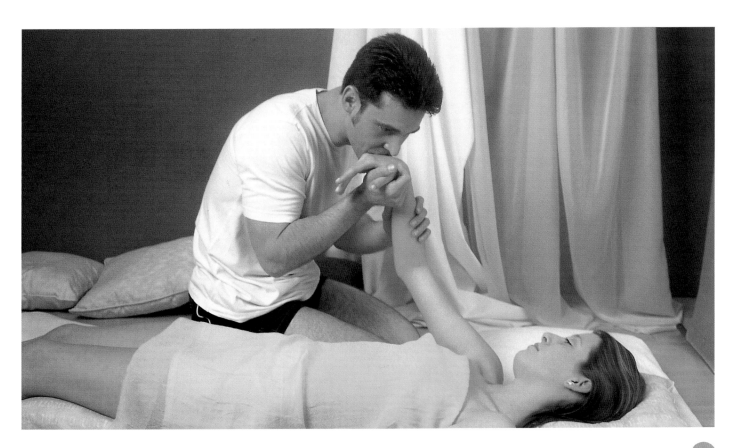

SENSUAL BACK MASSAGE

A back massage is a totally blissful and sensual experience. If your time is limited, this is an area you should definitely include. We all have knotted muscles somewhere in the back and shoulder area, which arise for a variety of reasons. Stress (physical and emotional), bad posture in our everyday activities (e.g. slouching over our desks), carrying children around or excessive gardening or sporting activities all take their toll.

Your lover should lie on his or her front with one pillow/cushion under the ankles to help the back to relax, and one under the head and shoulders. The arms should be placed comfortably at the sides. The body should be completely covered.

STEP 1   TUNING IN

Your initial contact is very important as it allows both you and your lover to release all tension and totally relax.

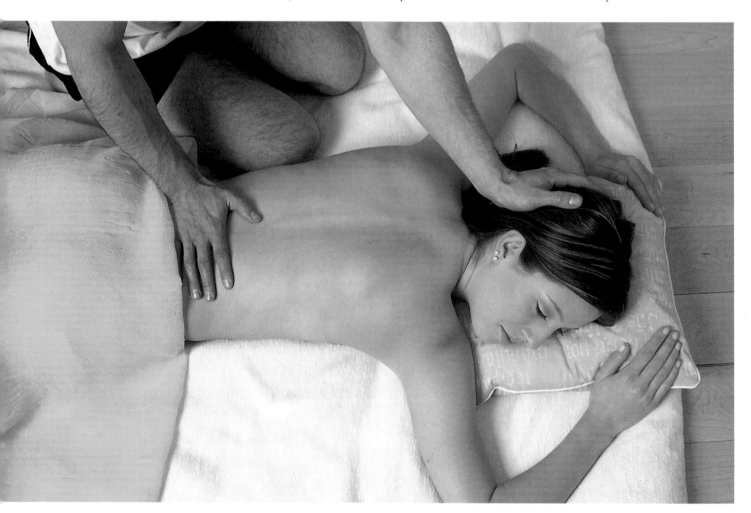

Position yourself at the side of your lover and lower your hands gently onto the back. One hand should rest gently on top of the head whilst the other hand rests at the base of the spine. Take a few deep breaths feeling the relaxation and allowing the healing energy to flow through the body. After a minute or so lift them gently off the body.

STEP 2 SPREADING THE OIL/LONG STROKING

Kneeling at the side of the waist, start to apply the oil using stroking movements. Place the palms of your relaxed hands at the bottom of the back, one hand either side of the spine with your fingers pointing towards the head.

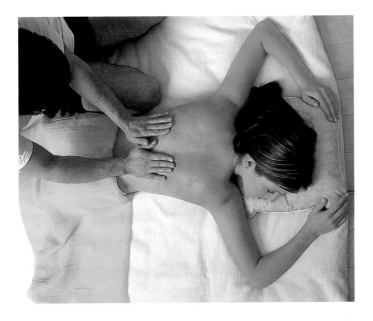

Stroke up the back towards the neck using your body weight to lean into the movement for a firmer pressure.

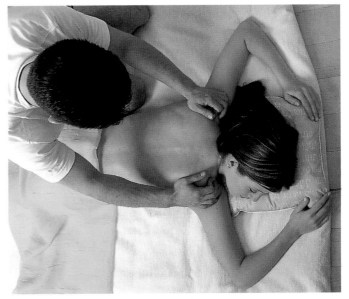

As your hands reach the top of the back, stroke out across the shoulders, molding your hands to the contours of the body.

Repeat these long stroking movements several times to establish your own rhythm and to accustom your lover to your hands.

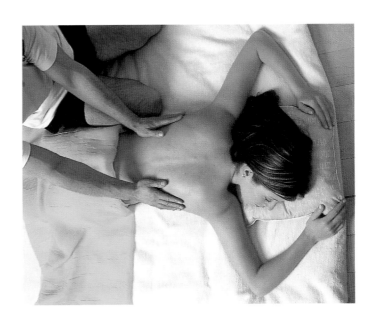

Allow your hands to glide gently back down the sides of the body with a feather-light touch.

STEP 3 ALTERNATE HANDS LONG STROKING

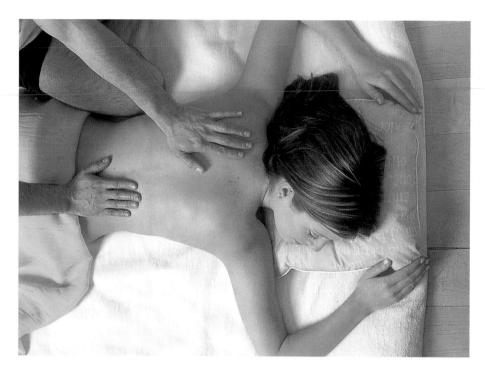

Place both hands palms down, one either side of the back, one hand on the lower back and one on the shoulder area, fingers pointing towards the head.

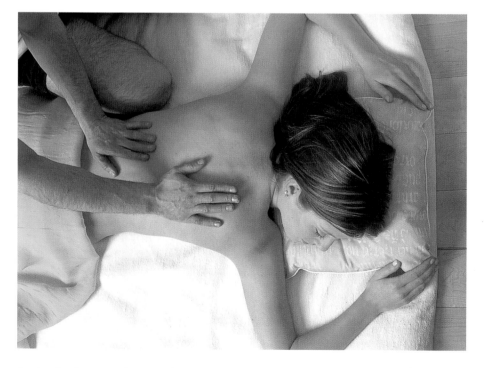

Stroke firmly upwards using the hand on the lower back whilst your upper hand glides down the spine. This movement feels wonderful and is excellent for loosening up the back.

STEP 4 CIRCLE STROKING

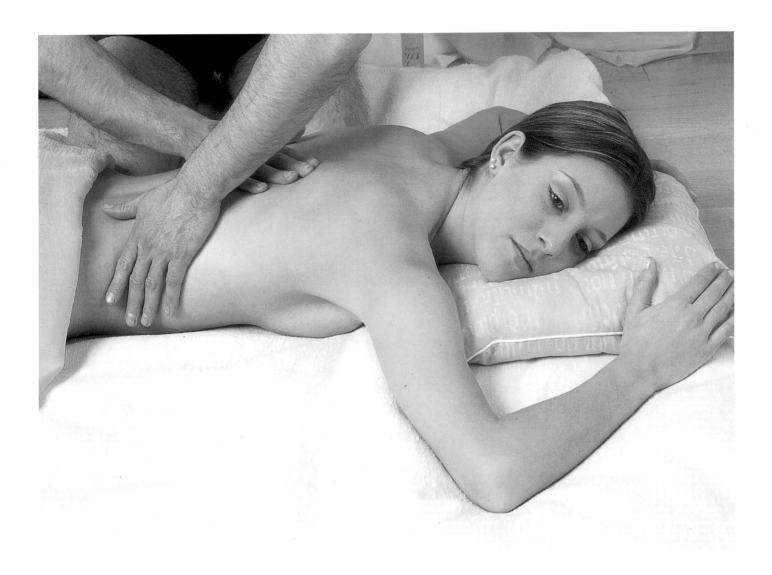

Position yourself to the side of your lover. Place both hands around the shoulder blade on the opposite side of the body.

As you complete a circle your hands will cross over. Although you will have to lift one hand over the other, ensure that you keep contact with one hand.

Using the whole of the palms of your hands make large stroking movements in a clockwise circular action with one hand following the other.

Now repeat these circular stroking movements on the side of the back nearest you.

STEP 5 STRETCHING THE BACK (HANDS)

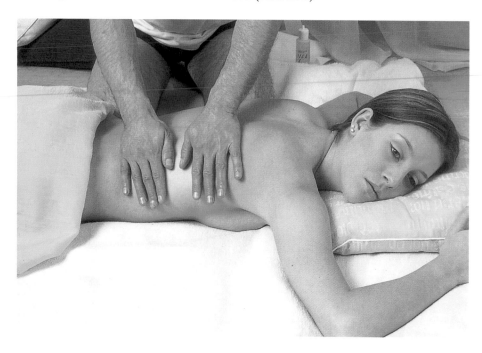

Place both hands palms down roughly in the center of the side of
the back furthest away from you.

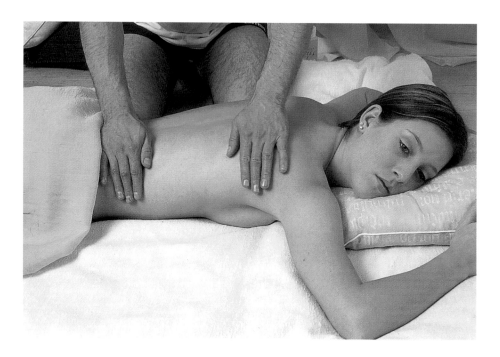

Gradually draw the hands away from each other with firm
pressure — one hand will slide up the back towards the head
whilst the other hand slides down towards the base of the spine.
Lean into the hands using your body weight for extra pressure.

Repeat on the side of the back nearest you.

STEP 6 STRETCHING THE BACK (FOREARMS)

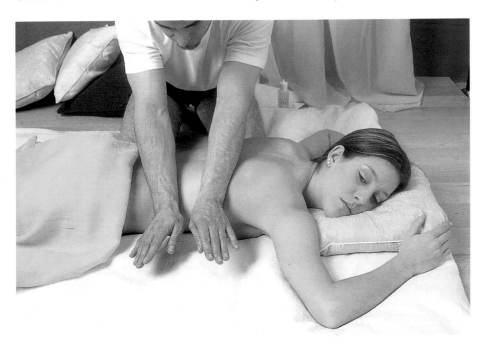

To really stretch the back, the forearms are an ideal tool. Place both forearms horizontally across the back on the side of the back furthest away from you.

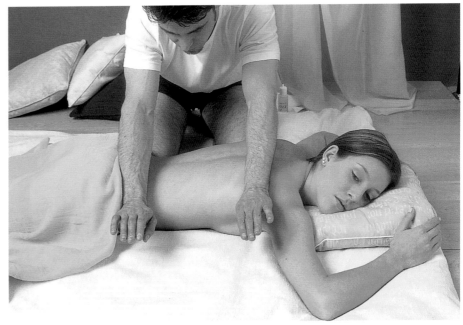

Gradually draw them apart so that one forearm glides up towards the neck, the other moves towards the buttocks. Then repeat on the side of the back nearest you.

STEP 7 PULLING UP THE SIDES OF THE BACK

Kneeling comfortably by the side of your lover facing the buttock area, place both hands on the far side of the back with your fingertips just touching the massage surface.

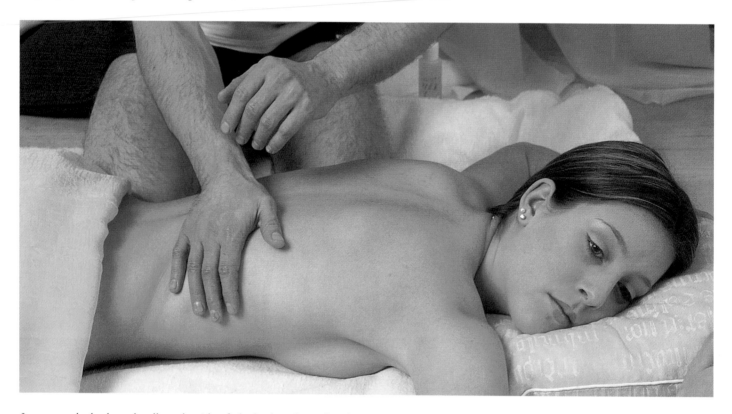

Lean over the body and pull up the side of the back with one hand.

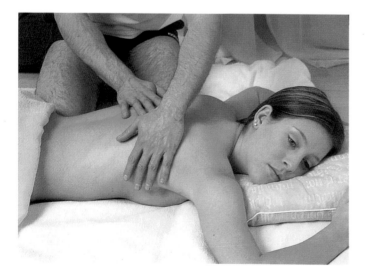

As this hand reaches the top of the back and lifts off, pull up the side with the other hand. As you pull up with your alternate hands, work up the back. When you reach the top of the back, work down the back.

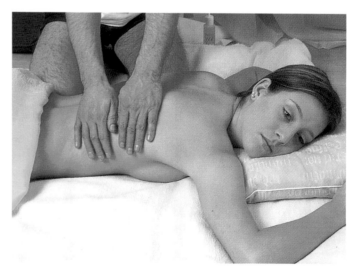

Now perform these movements pulling up with both hands at the same time.

The whole of step 7 should be repeated on the other side of the back.

STEP 8 KNEADING THE SIDES OF THE BACK

By this time your lover should be completely relaxed (possibly even asleep), and ready for some deeper sensual massage movements. Kneading is excellent for relaxing tight muscles and eliminating toxins. Position yourself at the side of the body facing the buttocks and place your hands down flat on the side of the back opposite you.

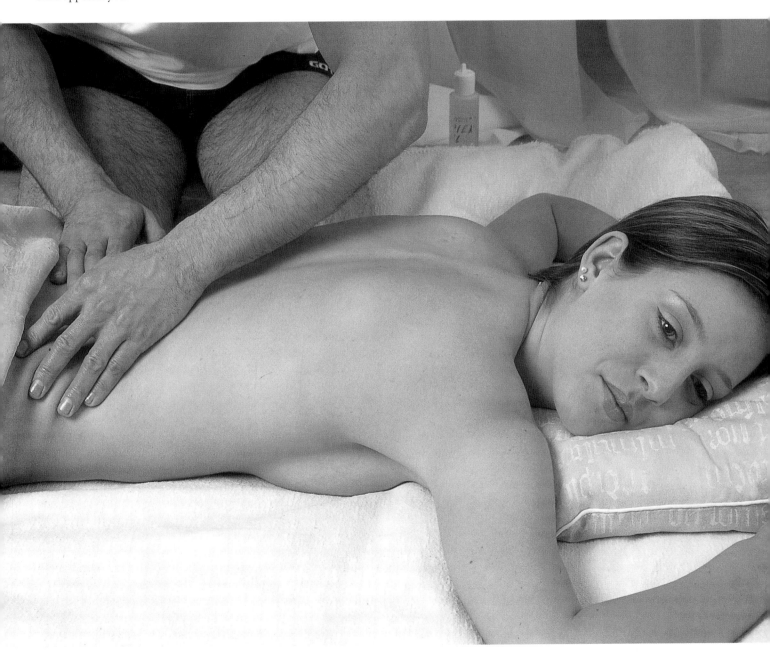

Starting at the buttock area, and using one hand, grasp and squeeze the muscle (not the skin) between your fingers and thumb and bring it up towards the other hand. As you release, use the other hand to grasp and squeeze a new handful of flesh.

As you work up the side of the back you will notice that this movement is much easier to perform around the fleshy waist area.

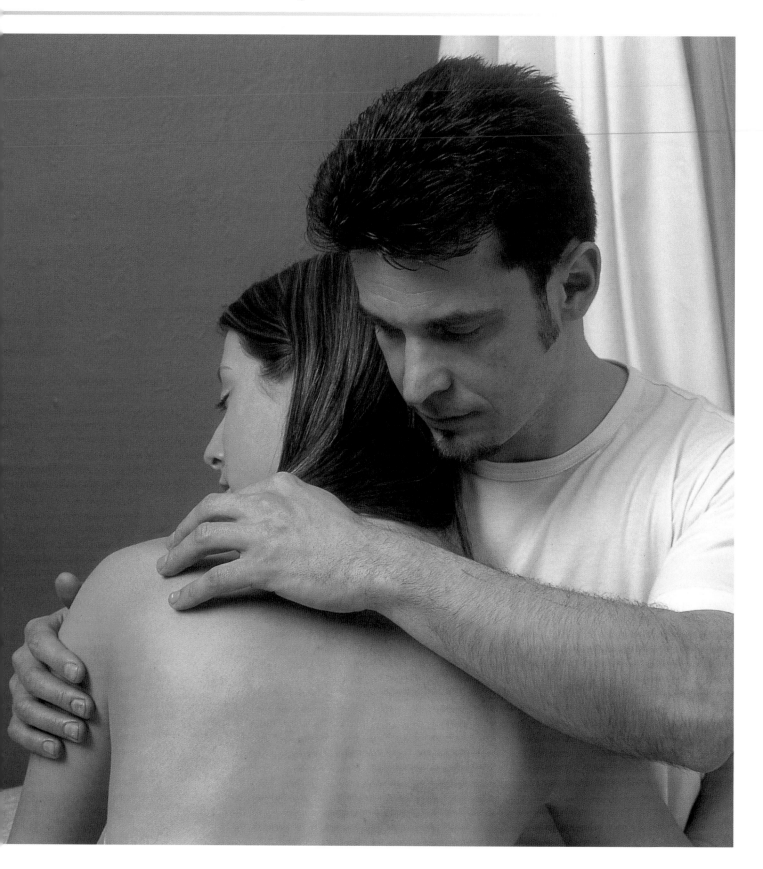

STEP 9 CIRCULAR THUMB PRESSURES
ON THE SPINAL MUSCLES

Now you are going to try to unravel the knots that build up so easily either side of the spine. This movement is most effective if you sit astride your lover although it is possible to work from the side if you prefer.

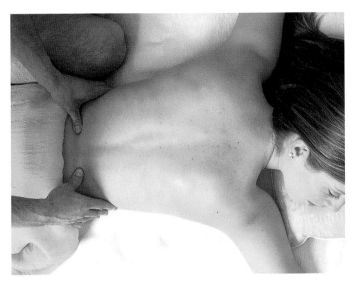

Look for two dimples at the base of the spine. Place the balls of your thumbs into these dimples.

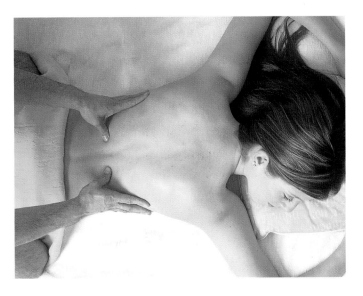

As you reach the base of the neck, allow your hands to glide back to the starting point with no pressure.

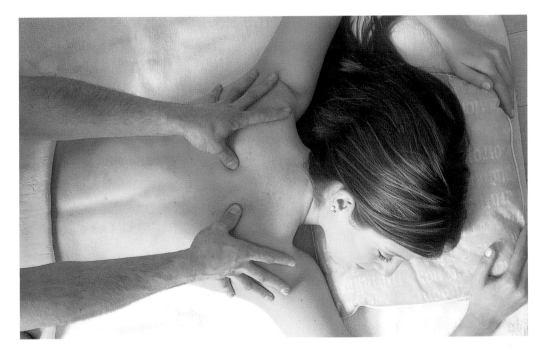

Make small, slow, firm outward circular movements with your thumbs travelling up towards the neck. Try to keep the thumbs parallel and the same distance apart as you work up the back.

If you come across any knots and nodules then try to gently break them down. You may either circle the thumbs outwards over the tight area or for deeper penetration place one thumb on top of the other and press slowly and deeply into the problem area.

STEP 10 PUSHING DOWN THE SIDES OF THE BACK

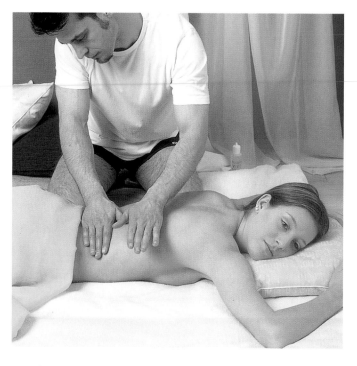

Kneel comfortably at the side of your lover and place both hands palms down on the opposite side of the back but NOT touching the spine.

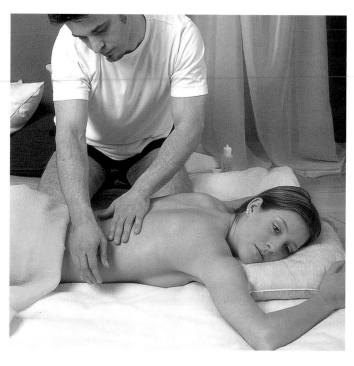

With alternate hands work up and down the back pushing downwards.

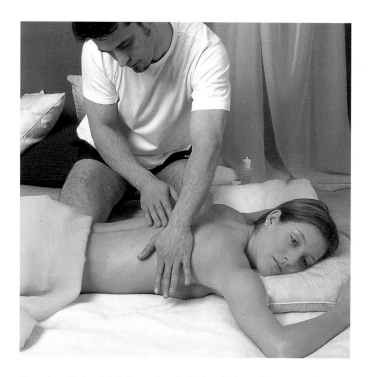

One hand should follow closely behind the other to establish a good rhythm.

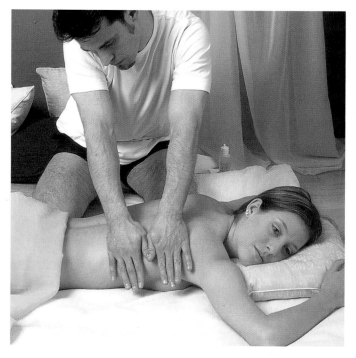

If you wish you may push down using both hands at once. These movements are soothing and help to take away any toxins that have been released around the spine.

THE BUTTOCKS

The buttocks hold in a lot of tension, which is easily released. They are also a very sensual area and contain many pressure points that can enhance sexual response.

STEP 11 CIRCULAR STROKING OF THE BUTTOCKS

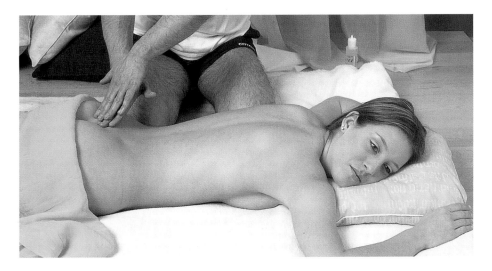

Position yourself at the side of your lover and place one hand flat on the top of the other on one of the buttocks. Make large figure-of-eight movements circling over one buttock and then over the other.

STEP 12 KNEADING THE BUTTOCKS

To knead the buttock muscles, place your hands palms downwards and pick up and squeeze the flesh with one hand and bring it towards you. Repeat with the other hand. Alternatively squeeze and release until the whole of the buttock area has been covered.

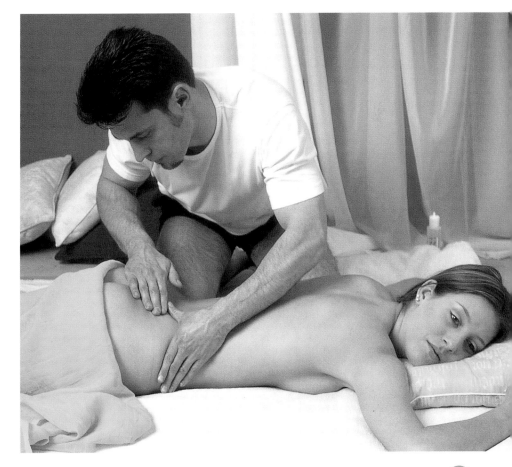

STEP 13 PRESSURES ON THE SEXUAL
 AROUSAL POINTS

STEP 14 KNUCKLING THE BUTTOCKS

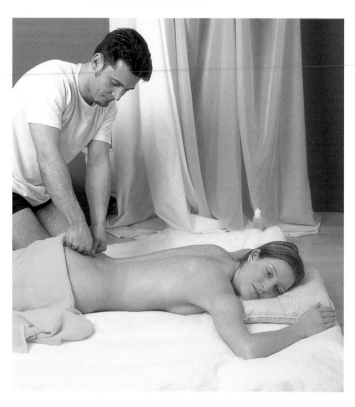

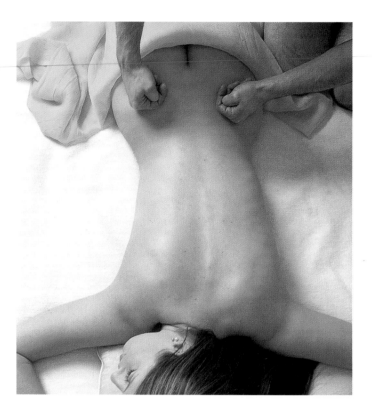

To increase sexual desire and vigor, commence just above the crease of the buttocks. Using very gentle pressure make small circular movements with one thumb on top of the other from the crease of the buttocks to the top of the buttocks, moving upwards in a straight line.

To perform this movement, make your hands into loose fists and place one fist onto each buttock. Rotate the middle section of your fingers around in a circular direction without taking your hands off the body. These knuckling movements disperse any remaining toxins and also ensure that all sexual arousal points have been massaged.

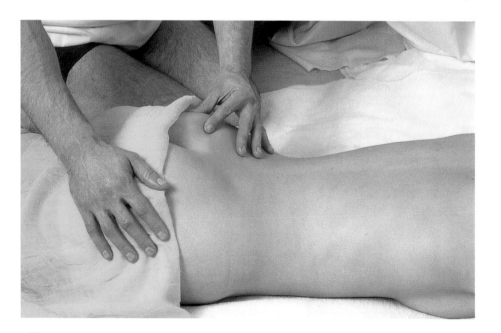

STEP 15 PLUCKING
THE BUTTOCKS

Plucking is a very sensual movement when performed over the buttocks and has the added benefit of helping to tone and keep them in shape. Place both hands palms down onto the buttocks. Gently pick up small areas of flesh between your thumbs and fingers and let them slip through your hands.

THE NECK AND SHOULDERS

There is always tightness and stiffness in this area. It is very common to hunch the shoulders or let them roll forward. Tension in the neck area is also usually present and often gives rise to headaches and migraine.

STEP 16 CIRCLING BOTH SHOULDER BLADES

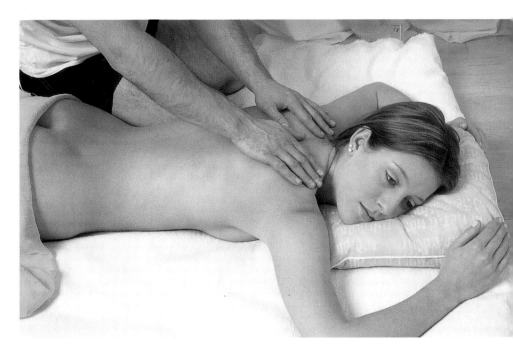

Place one hand palm down on the right shoulder blade and your other hand on the left shoulder blade.

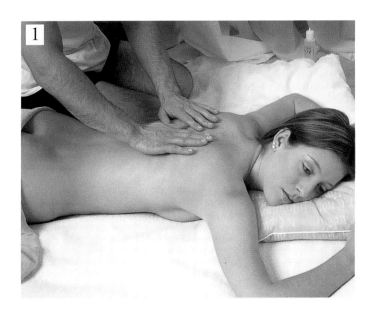
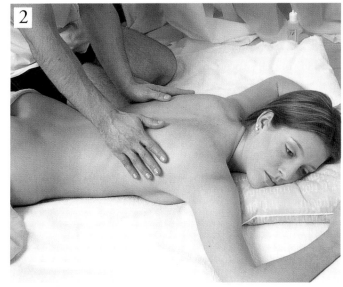

Make large outward circles with both hands simultaneously.(1, 2)

STEP 17 CIRCLING THE SHOULDER, ONE HAND ON TOP OF THE OTHER

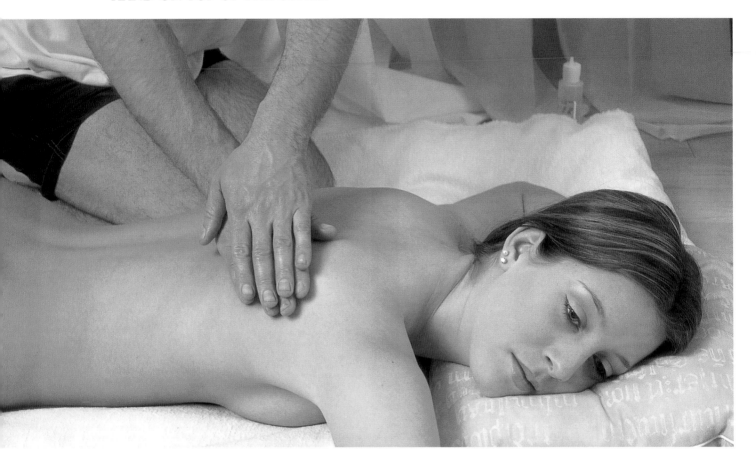

Position yourself at the side of your lover. Place one hand flat on top of the other hand and using the whole of the hand make large circular movements on and around the shoulder blade opposite you.

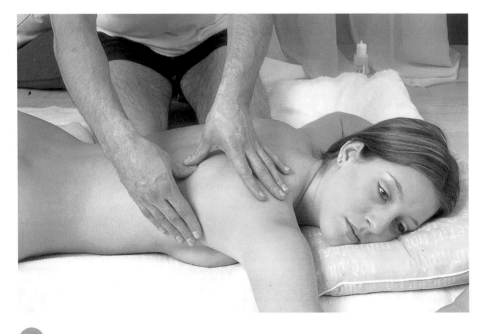

STEP 18 THUMB PRESSURES AROUND THE SHOULDER BLADE

Now that you have warmed and loosened the area, you are going to work deeper to dispel the tension which builds up around the shoulder blade. Still working on the shoulder opposite you, place the balls of your thumbs at the bottom of the shoulder blade and make small circular movements around it, gradually working up to the top.

Repeat steps 17 and 18 on the other shoulder blade.

STEP 19 KNEADING THE SHOULDERS

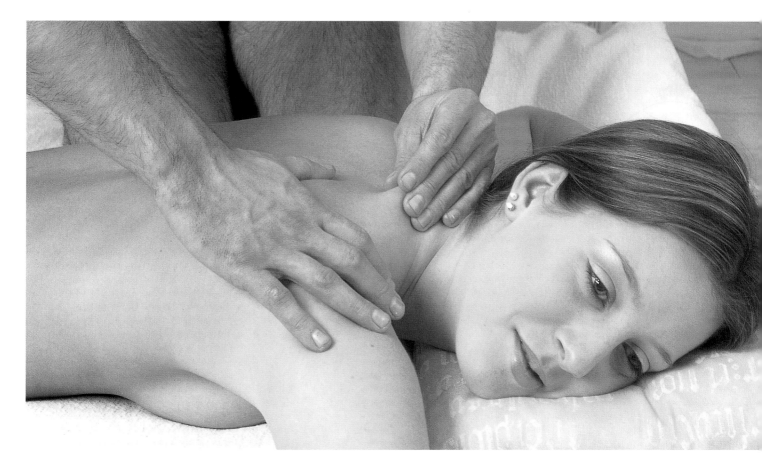

Work across the top of the shoulders rhythmically squeezing and bringing the flesh towards you with alternate hands.

STEP 20 KNEADING THE NECK

Ask your lover to place their forehead onto their hands to straighten out the back of the neck. Place both hands flat down molding them to the contours of the neck. Very GENTLY pick up and squeeze the neck muscles, making sure that you are using the whole of your hands and not just your fingers, which can pinch.

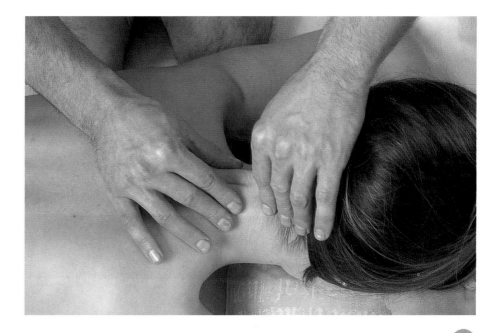

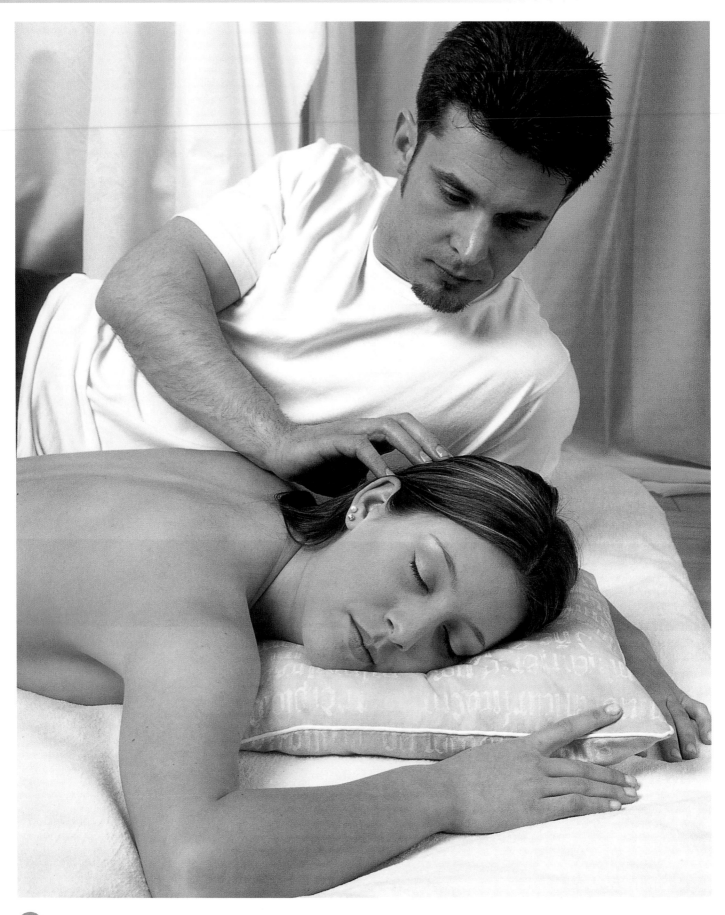

STEP 21 LONG STROKING THE WHOLE BACK

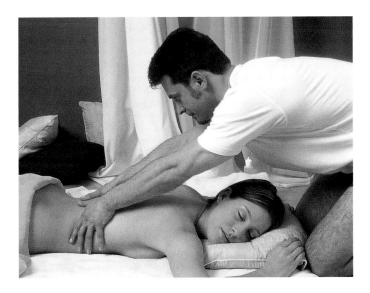

Position yourself at your lover's head in a comfortable kneeling position. Place your hands palms down at the top of the shoulders. Stroke the entire back moving downwards and over the buttocks. Allow your hands to glide back to your starting point with no pressure.

STEP 22 DIAGONAL STROKING

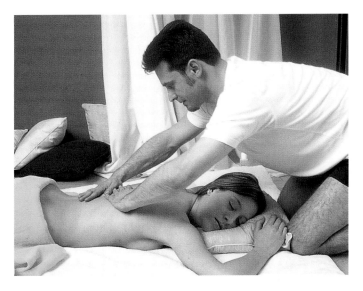

Still kneeling at your lover's head, allow your hands, palms facing downward, to rest crossed one on top of the other at the base of the neck. Move them slowly away from each other in opposite directions so that by the time they reach the sides of the body your hands are making a 'V'. Slowly glide them back together again and repeat this movement until you reach the buttocks. You may also work from the buttocks up towards the neck.

STEP 23 CAT STROKING

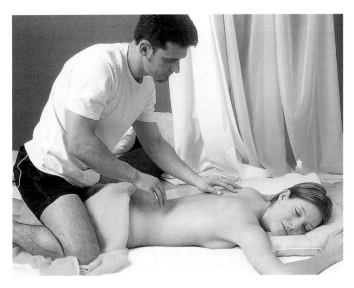

Position yourself at the side of your lover near the buttocks or sit astride him/her. Place your right hand palm downward at the base of the neck and stroke slowly down the back using almost no pressure. As your right hand reaches the buttocks, lift it off and repeat the movement with your left hand. Repeat these movements several times, one hand following the other. It should feel like one continuous movement.

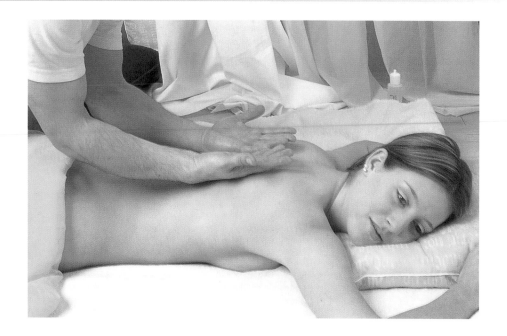

STEP 24
STROKING WITH THE BACK OF THE HANDS

Place the backs of both hands at the top of the body, one either side of the spine, and stroke them gently down towards the buttocks. Then glide the backs of your hands upward to your starting position, moving along the sides of the body.

STEP 25
THE FINAL TOUCH
FINGERTIP STROKING

Working from the side close to the buttocks or sitting astride your lover stroke down the back very slowly using just the fingertips so that you are barely touching the skin.

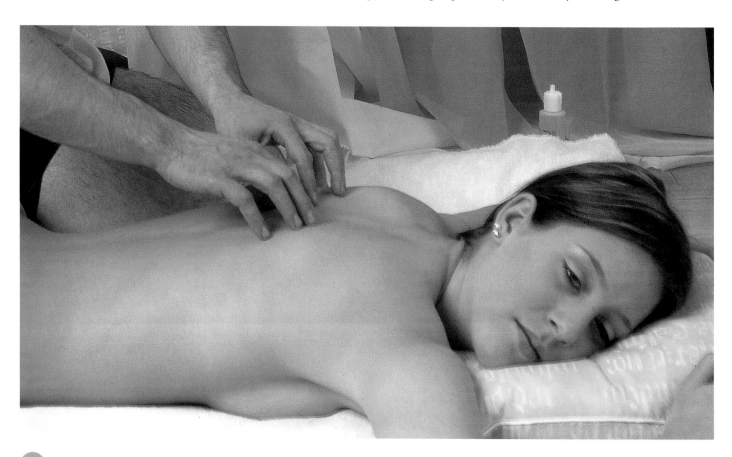

SENSUAL MASSAGE OF THE BACK OF THE LEG

Leg massage is very beneficial as it improves the circulation, helps to prevent varicose veins, relieves tightness and cramp in the muscles, reduces swelling in the lower leg and ankles and counteracts cellulite. It is also very sensual particularly the inner area of the thigh. This section describes just a few movements that are useful for the legs.

STEP 1 TUNING INTO THE LEGS

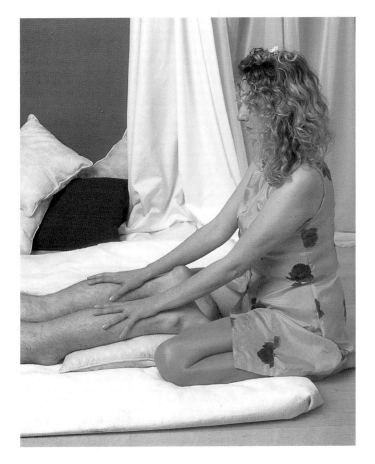

Kneel at your lover's feet and rest the palms of your hands gently, one on each leg. Take a few deep breaths until you feel the tension melting away.

STEP 2 LONG STROKING ON BOTH LEGS

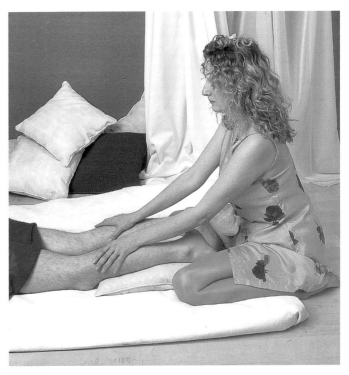

Place the palms of both hands at the backs of both ankles. Stroke up both legs from the ankles to the buttocks, molding your hands to the contours of the legs.

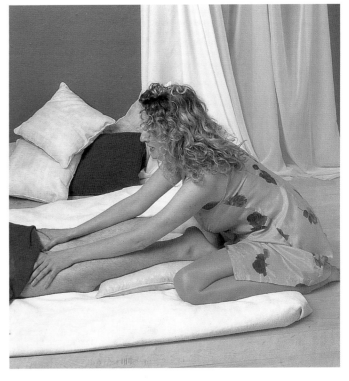

Glide back down the legs with a feather-light touch.

STEP 3   KNEADING THE LEG

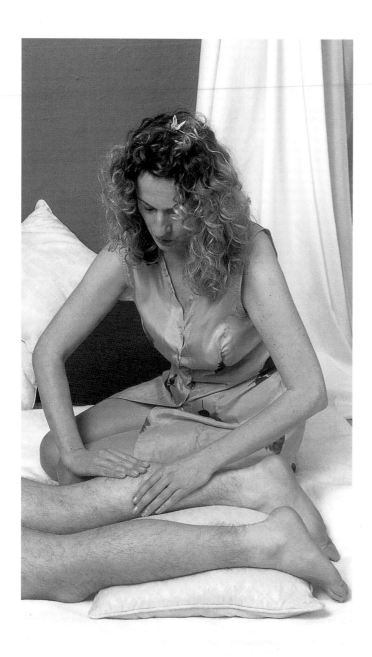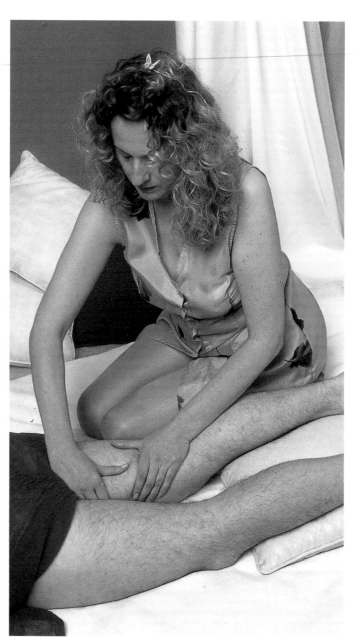

Position yourself at your lover's side and place both hands flat down on the calf muscles. With one hand grasp and squeeze the muscle (not the skin) and bring it towards the other hand. As you release, use the other hand to grasp a new handful of flesh.

Alternately squeeze and release bunches of flesh, working all over the calf and thigh. Maintain a slow rhythm for deep relaxation.

STEP 4 ALTERNATE HEEL OF HAND STROKING UP THE BACK OF THE LEG

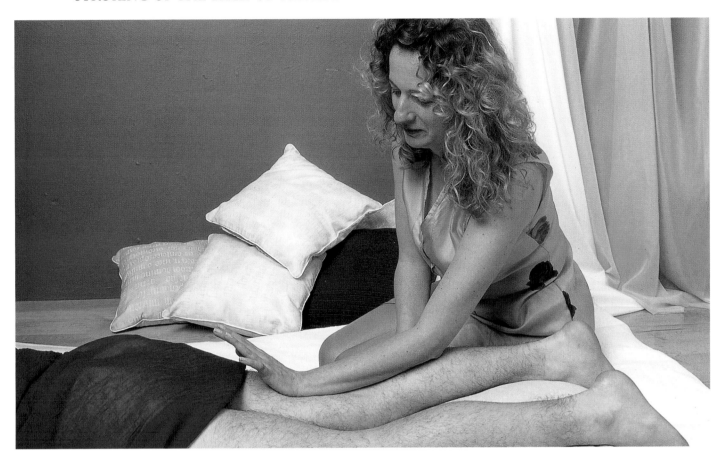

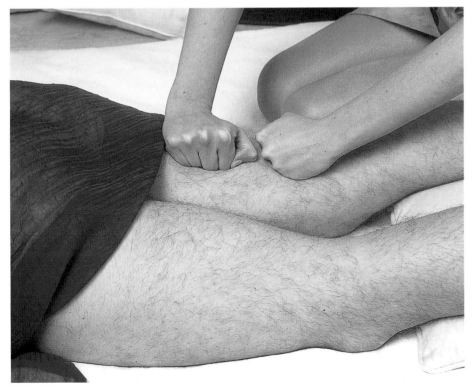

Place the heels of your hands just above the back of the knee. (Do not press into the back of the knee, as this is a very delicate area). Push one hand firmly into the back of the thigh working up the leg, and then push with your other hand. Allow the heels of your hands to move alternately up the back of the thigh.

STEP 5 KNUCKLING THE THIGH

If the legs are very congested or obstinate cellulite is present, then some deeper movements will be required. Make your hands into loose fists and place them onto the thigh. Rotate your fists in a circular direction to break down and eliminate the fatty deposits.

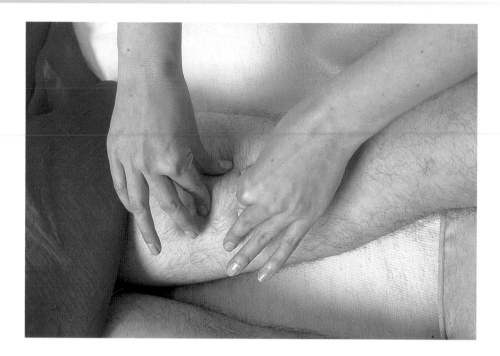

STEP 6 PLUCKING THE THIGH

Place both hands, palms down, onto a fleshy area of the thigh and gently pick up small areas of flesh between your thumbs and fingers. Let these slip through your hands.

STEP 7 THE FINAL TOUCH —
ALTERNATE FINGERTIP STROKING

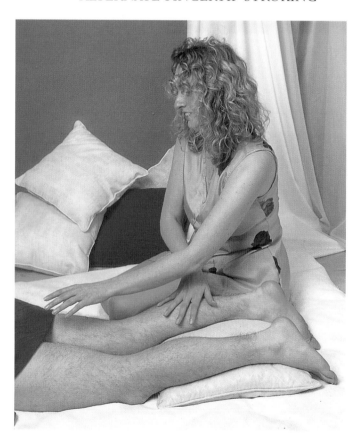

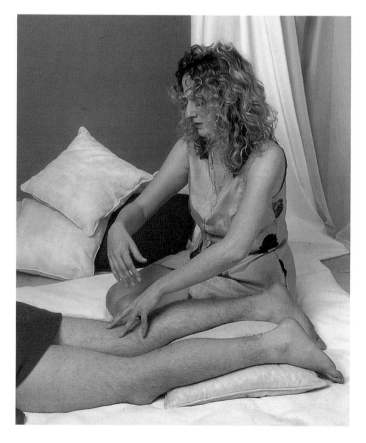

Starting at the top of the thigh, stroke slowly down the leg using just the fingertips of one hand so that you are barely touching the skin.

As your first hand reaches the ankle, lift it off gently as your other hand commences the stroking. Repeat steps 3 to 7 on the other leg.

FRONT OF THE BODY

Ask your lover to turn over. Place cushions/pillows under their head and another under their knees for maximum comfort.

STEP 1   GREETING AND STROKING THE FOOT

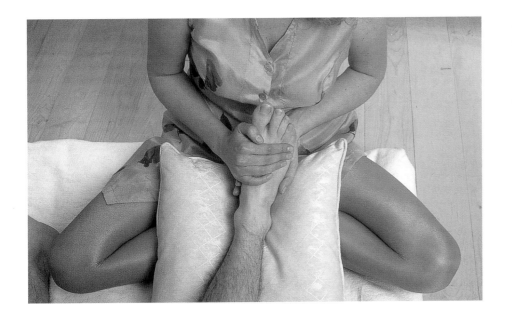

SENSUAL MASSAGE OF THE FOOT AND FRONT OF THE LEG

The foot is a very sensual area. According to reflexology the feet precisely mirror the body. All the organs and parts of the body are found in miniature on the feet and therefore as you massage you will be affecting the whole body and not just the feet.

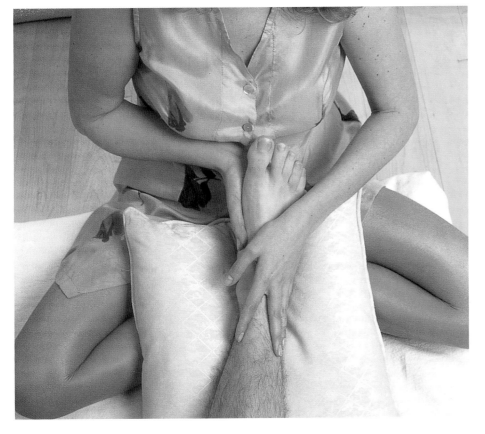

Only a minute amount of oil is required to work on the feet. Too much lubricant will make it difficult for you to hold the foot properly and will cause your fingers to slip and slide around. Clasp the foot gently between both hands to tune in.

Using both hands, stroke the whole foot firmly to avoid tickling. Cover the top, sides and sole of the foot. Work up from the toes, gliding around the anklebones and back again. Repeat several times to thoroughly relax the foot and to help disperse any excess fluid, especially around the ankles.

STEP 2 KNEADING THE FOOT

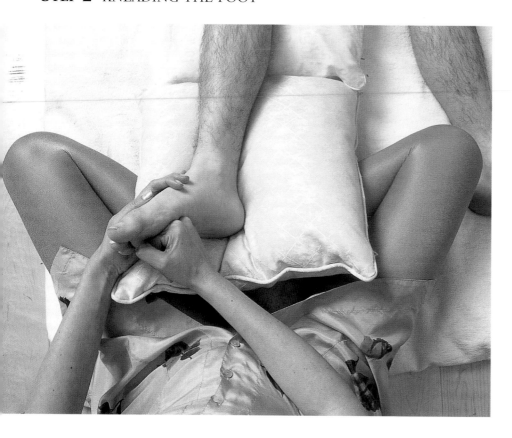

Wrap one hand around the foot with thumb on the sole, fingers on the top. Make a fist with your other hand and place it on the fleshy area on the ball of the foot. Using a gentle circular motion, work from the ball of the foot to the heel.

STEP 3 SPREADING THE FOOT

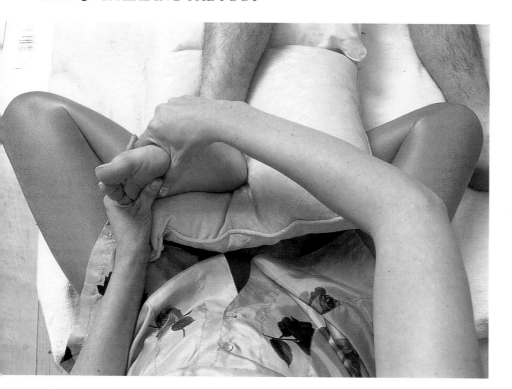

Holding the foot with both hands, place the thumbs on the sole, with your fingers resting on the top of the foot — one hand should be slightly higher than the other. Pull the thumbs away and past each other towards the edges of the foot and then allow them to glide back towards each other. Work the thumbs in this zigzag fashion from the base of the toes to the heels and back again, feeling as if you are opening out the foot.

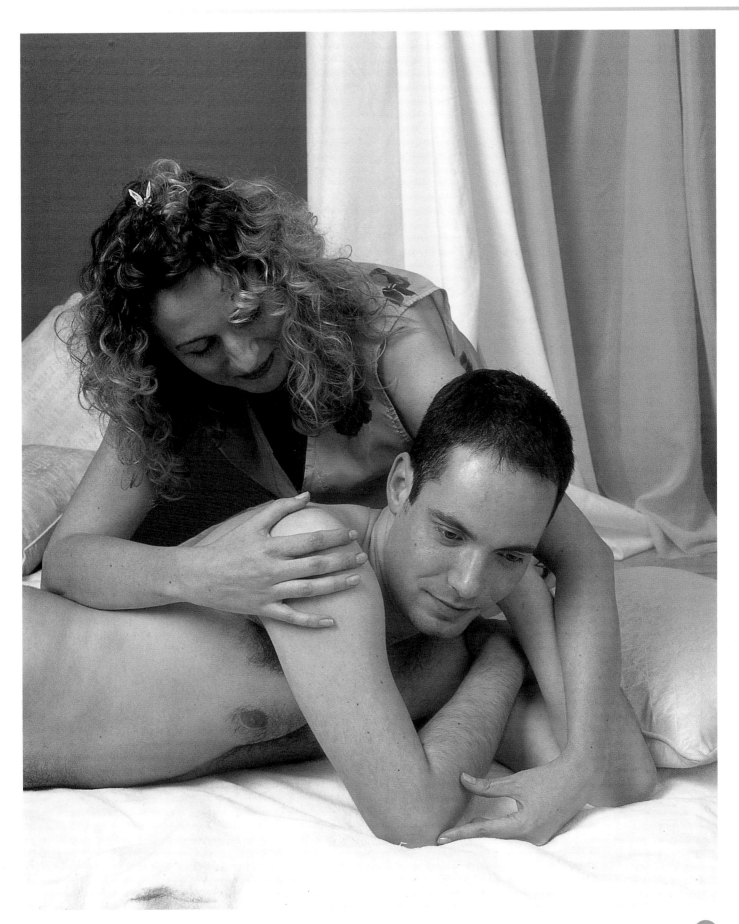

STEP 4 PUSH AND PULL THE FOOT

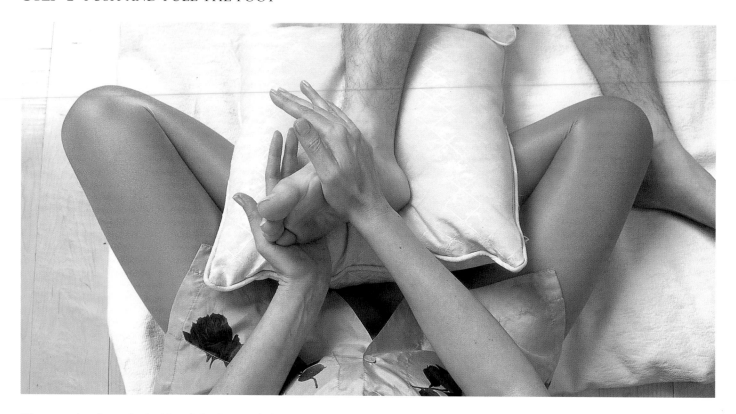

Place one hand on the inside of the foot and the other on the outside. Using the heels of your hands, pull the outside of the foot towards you with one hand as you push the inside of the foot away from you and vice versa. Work along the edges of the foot from the heel to the toes and back down again.

STEP 5 TOE LOOSENING

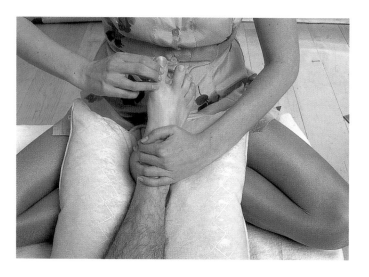

Support the foot in one hand, thumb on the sole of the foot, fingers wrapped around the top. Using your thumb and index finger, gently stretch and rotate each toe both clockwise and counter-clockwise.

STEP 6 FREEING THE ANKLE

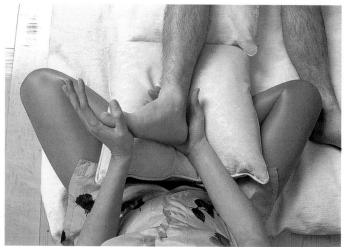

Cup the heel in one hand grasping the top of the foot with your other hand. Slowly and gently rotate the ankle first in one direction and then in the other.

STEP 7 LONG STROKING OF THE FRONT LEG

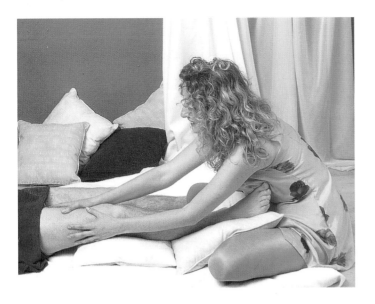

Stroke up the leg from the ankle to the top of the thigh using only light pressure over the knee. As your hands reach the top of the thigh, glide them gently down the sides.

STEP 8 KNEADING THE THIGH

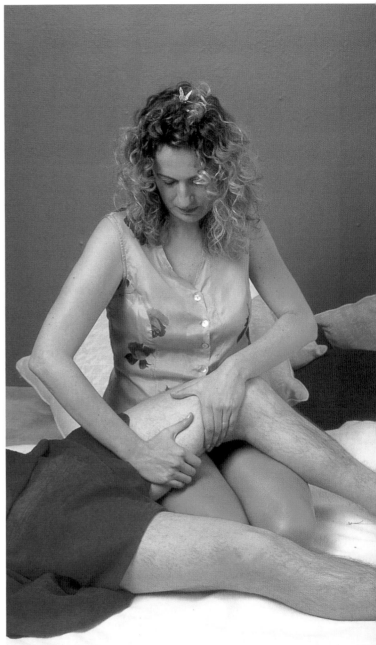

Knead the thigh muscles by squeezing and bringing the flesh towards you using alternate hands.

STEP 9 CIRCULAR THUMB PRESSURES ON
THE THIGH

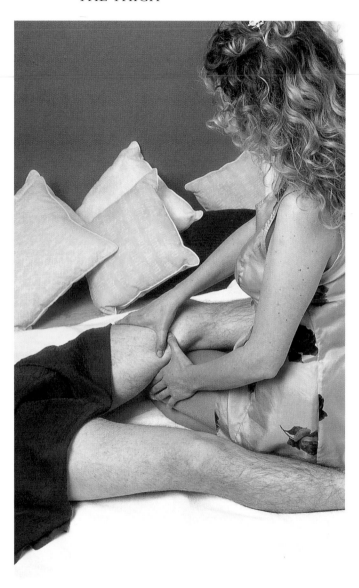

Sexual arousal points are very prevalent along the inner thigh area. This area will certainly excite your lover. Place the balls of the thumbs just above the knee on the inner aspect of the thigh. Make small circular movements with your thumbs until you reach the pubic area.

STEP 10 THE FINAL TOUCH — FINGERTIP
STROKING

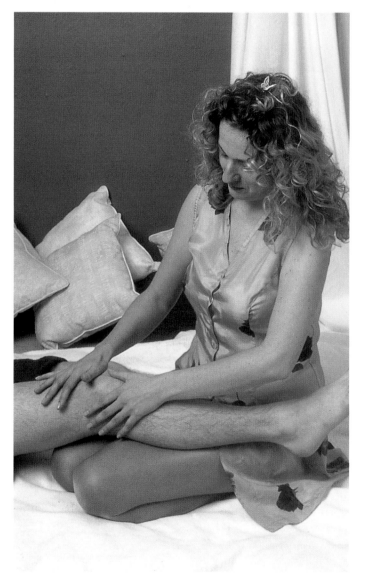

Place both hands, fingertips down, at the top of the thigh. With both hands stroke down the leg using just your fingertips. Very erotic.

Repeat all steps on the other foot and the front of the leg

SENSUAL ABDOMINAL MASSAGE

To have the abdomen massaged is a wonderful experience. It is very relaxing and soothes away the tension, which many people carry there. Digestive problems such as constipation and indigestion as well as menstrual problems benefit from a gentle abdominal massage and there are also many sensual stimulation points in this area.

STEP 1 TUNING IN

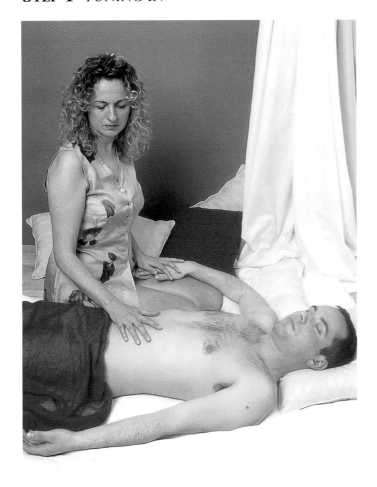

Kneel comfortably by the side of your lover. Lower both hands gently down to rest on top of the navel, and take a few deep breaths. Alternatively, you may prefer to rest one of your hands lightly on your lover's hand. As you do this you will probably notice your lover's breathing starting to deepen.

STEP 2 CIRCLING THE NAVEL

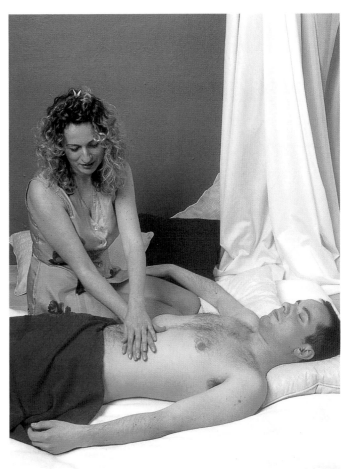

Employing very gentle, sensitive pressure, start to circle the navel moving in a clockwise direction. Gradually increase the size of your circles so that you encompass the whole of the abdomen.

STEP 3 CIRCLE STROKING

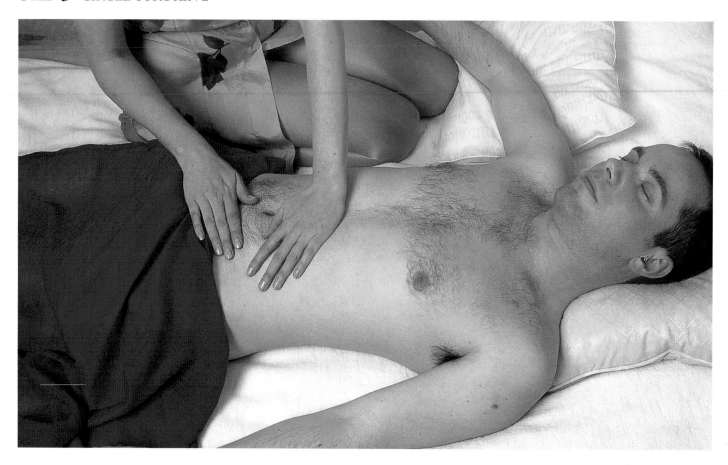

Place your hands flat down on the abdomen and perform circular stroking movements in a clockwise direction using both hands at the same time, one hand following behind the other. It should feel like one continuous circle if it is performed correctly.

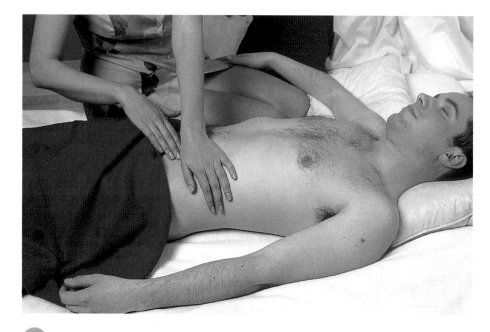

STEP 4 PULLING

Place both hands on your lover's far side with your fingertips touching the massage surface. Lean over the body and with one hand stroke gently and slowly up the side of the waist until you reach the navel. As your first hand lifts off, repeat the movement with your other hand. Cover the whole of the side of the abdomen with these pulling movements.

To work on the side nearest you, you may go to the other side of your lover if you find it awkward.

STEP 5 KNEADING

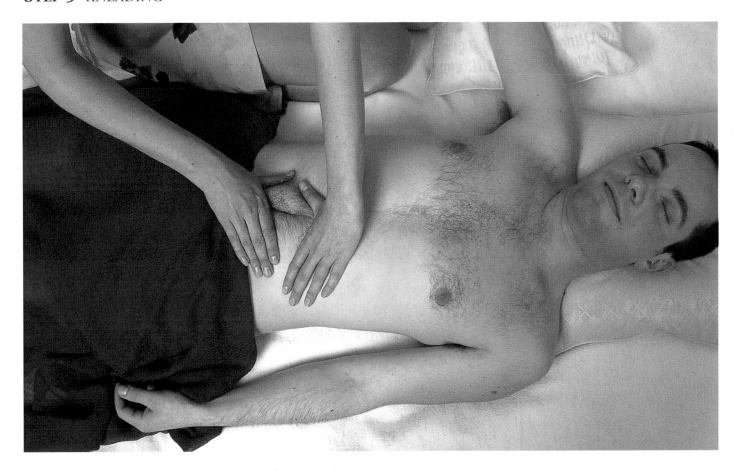

Alternately squeeze and release the flesh around the waist and hip area opposite you — there is usually plenty to grasp hold of. Then knead the side nearest you.

STEP 6 THE FINAL TOUCH — FINGERTIP CIRCULAR STROKING

With a feather light touch, stroke the abdomen in a clockwise direction barely touching the body with your fingertips. Gradually lift them very slowly away from the body.

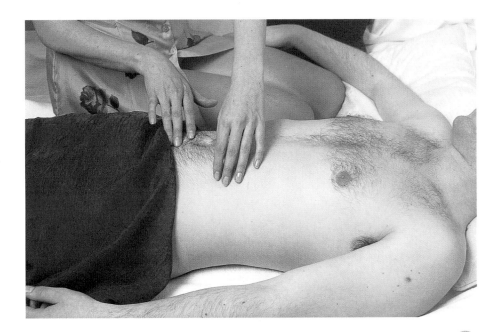

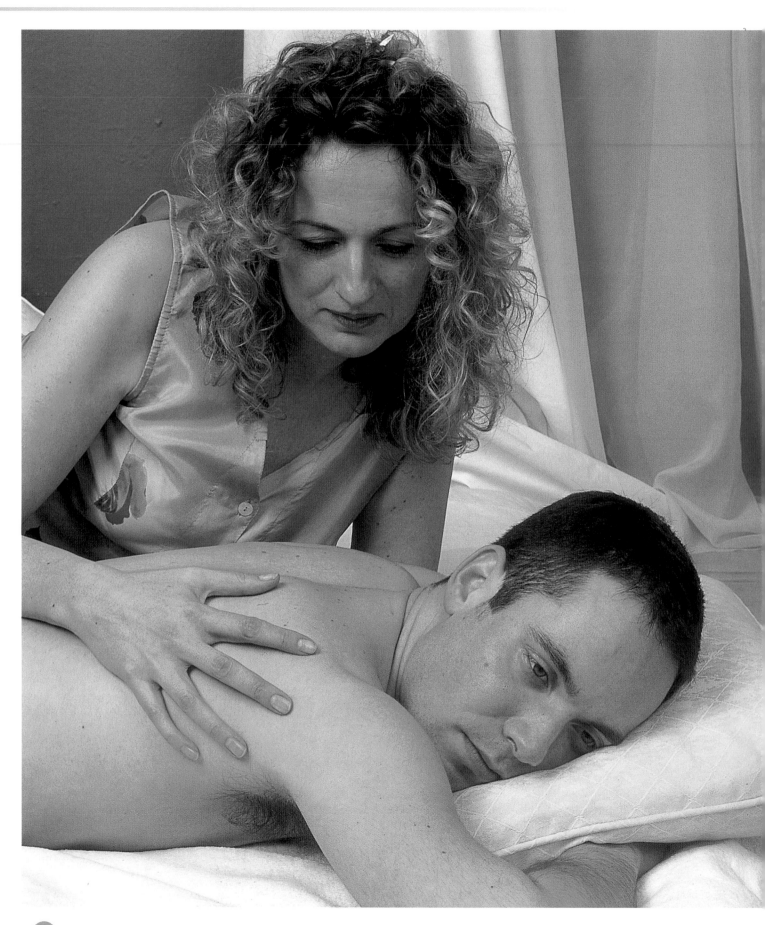

SENSUAL MASSAGE OF THE ARM AND HAND

Our arms and hands are in constant use throughout the day and are prone to many problems. A lot of emotion is expressed through our arms and hands. We show love and compassion to others by embracing them. We use our hands and arms to comfort our friends and express ourselves more clearly. Negative emotions such as anger and frustration can also be expressed for instance by shaking our fists. Massaging this area can therefore help to release pent-up emotions. Our general health is also affected when we massage the hands — according to hand reflexology they are a mini-map of the body and by massaging the reflex zones we are improving the health of the whole body.

STEP 1   TUNING IN

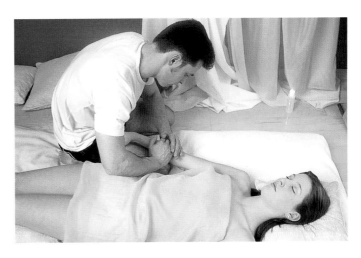

Kneel down at the side of your lover, and allow both hands to rest gently on their arm. Take a few deep breaths and feel the tension in the arm and hand releasing.

STEP 2 STROKING THE ARM

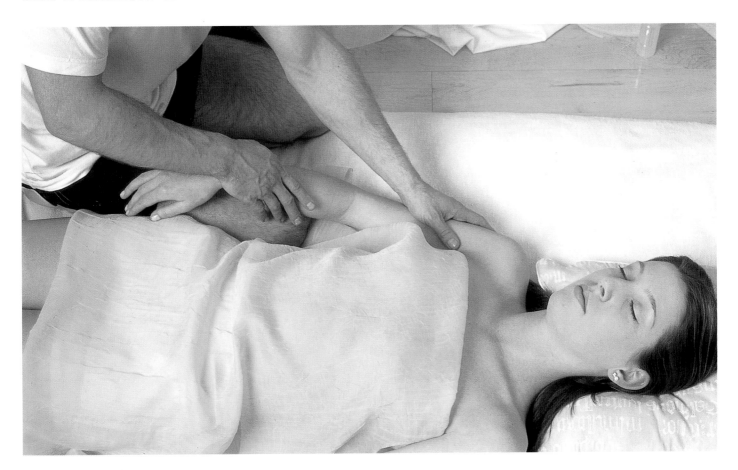

Place cupped hands across your lover's wrist and stroke up the arm from the wrist to the shoulder. When you reach the top of the arm, open out your hands and glide back down the sides with no pressure.

STEP 3 KNEADING THE UPPER ARM

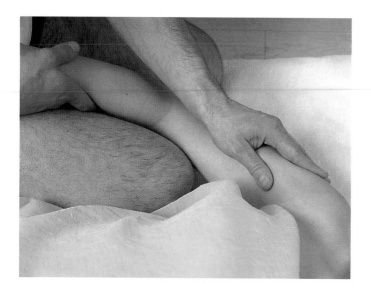

Using both hands, knead the muscles of the upper arm.

STEP 4 KNEADING THE FOREARM

Rest your lover's hand on your thigh. Support the wrist with one hand and gently knead the forearm with your other hand from the wrist to the elbow.

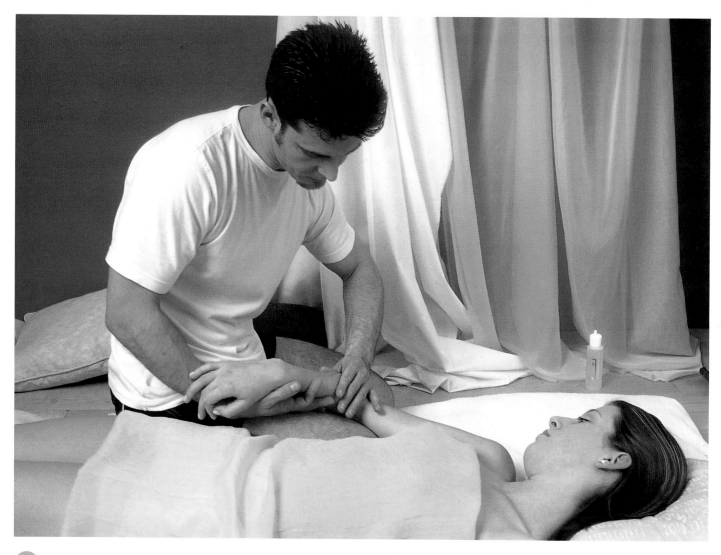

STEP 5 LOOSENING THE WRIST

Support the hand with your fingers and use your thumbs to gently massage in small circles all around the inside of the wrist.

Then turn the hand over and work in the same way on the other side.

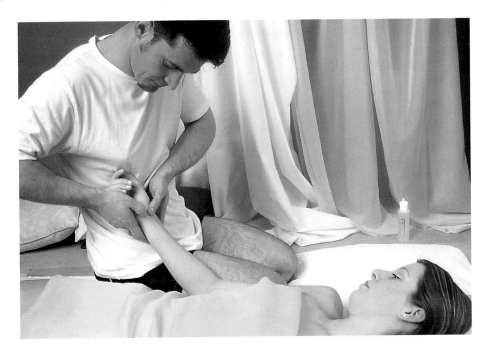

STEP 6 MOVING THE WRIST

Interlock your fingers with your lover and then gently and slowly rotate the wrist clockwise and counter-clockwise.

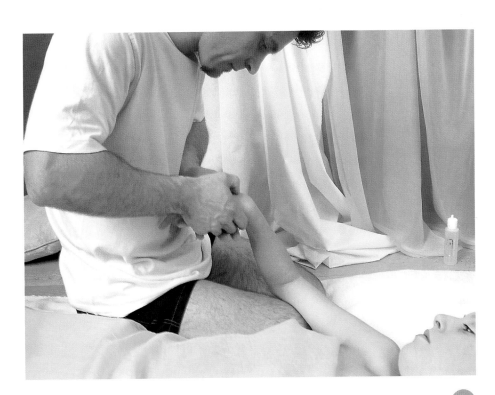

STEP 7 STROKING THE HANDS

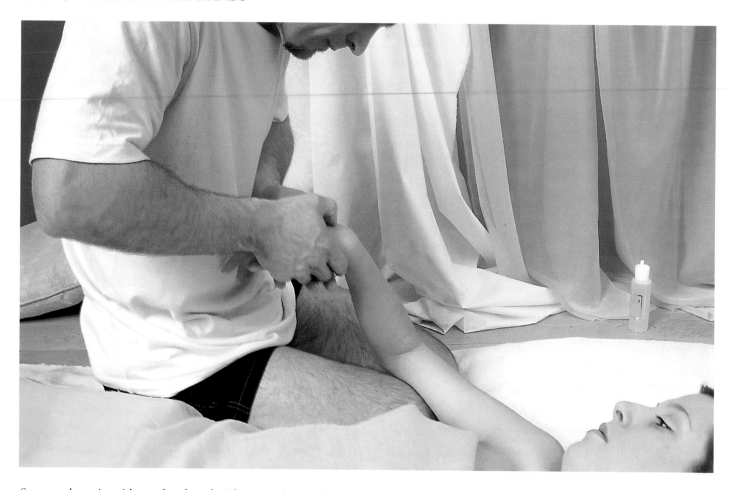

Support the wrist with one hand, and with your other hand stroke up to the top of the hand. These stroking movements should be performed on both sides of the hand.

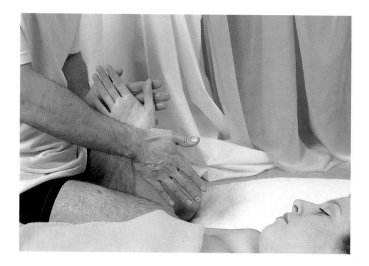

For a deeper movement on the palm you can use the heel of your hand.

STEP 8 OPENING THE HANDS

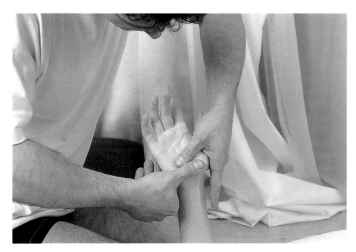

Take your lover's hand palm uppermost in both of yours, with both your thumbs flat in the center of the palm, fingers underneath.

STEP 9 STRETCH AND SQUEEZE THE FINGERS AND THUMBS

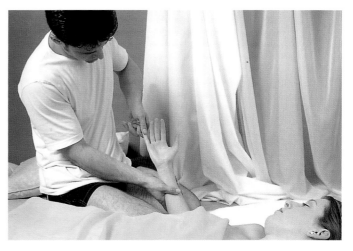

Hold your lover's wrist with one hand and gently and slowly stretch and squeeze each finger individually.

STEP 10 CIRCLING

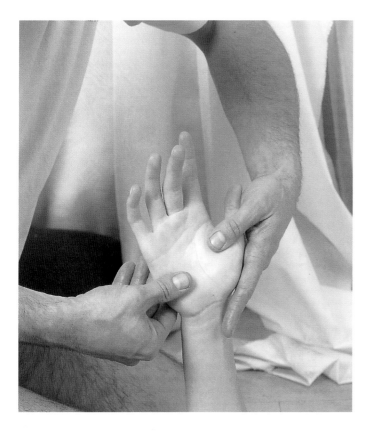

Slide your thumbs out to the side to gently open up the palm of the hand.

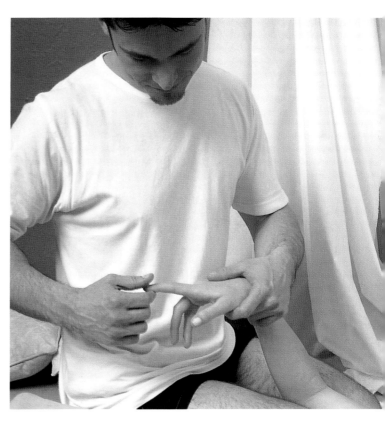

Circle the fingers and thumb individually both clockwise and counter-clockwise.

STEP 11 FINGERTIP STROKING OF THE HAND

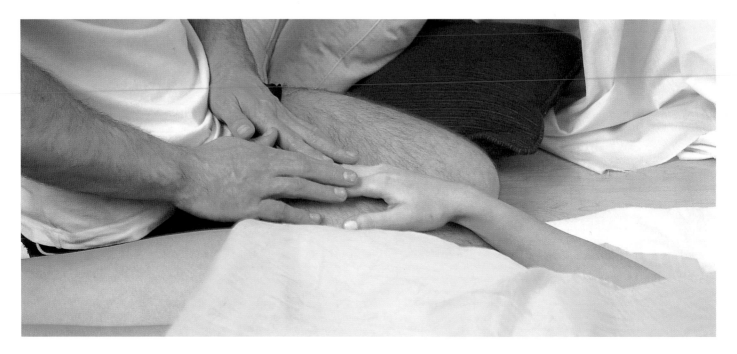

Using just your fingertips, stroke the hand gently from the wrist to the tips.

STEP 12 THE FINAL TOUCH — STROKING THE ARM

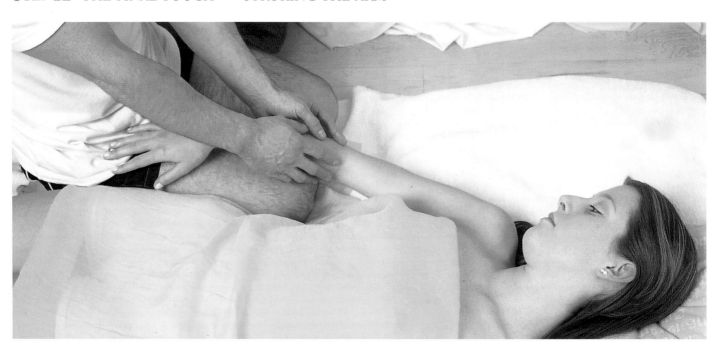

Stroke down the whole arm and hand using both hands together with the lightest of movements. On your final stroke, clasp your lover's hand between both your hands and gently squeeze it.

Repeat all steps on the other arm and hand.

SENSUAL MASSAGE OF THE CHEST AND NECK

The chest area is often very tight and congested due to bad posture or incorrect breathing (most people breathe from the chest instead of from the abdomen). Emotional problems are often stored in the chest area — hence the expression 'get it off your chest.' Massage of this area helps to release pent-up emotions and allows the chest to open up and relax.

Tightness in the neck is a very common problem and can lead to symptoms such as headaches, which can be relieved with massage.

STEP 1 TUNING IN

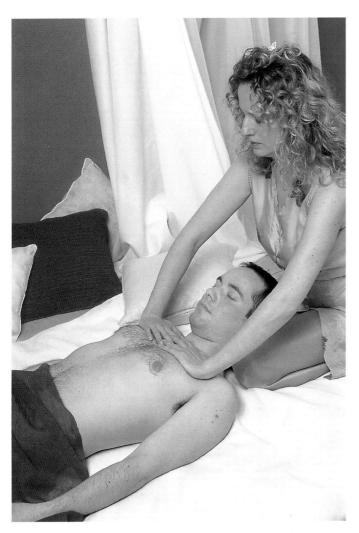

Kneel down behind your lover's head. Allow both hands to rest gently on your lover's shoulders and take a few deep breaths.

STEP 2 OPENING UP THE CHEST

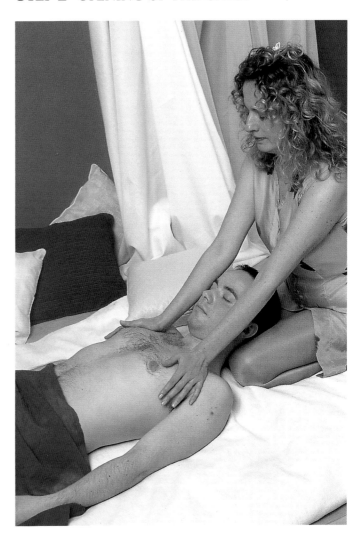

Place your hands, palms down, in the centre of the chest, with the fingertips facing towards each other. Stroke from the centre of the chest outwards and then stroke over the shoulders. Glide your hands back to your starting point with no pressure.

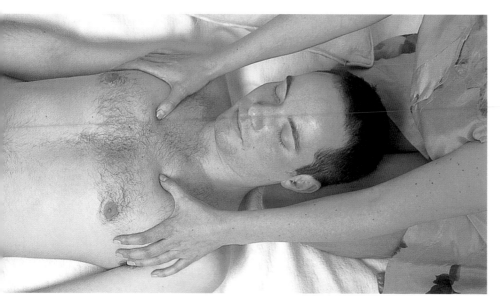

STEP 3 CIRCULAR PRESSURES

Place both thumbs in the center of the chest just below the collarbones and make small gentle circular movements with your thumbs. Work along the line of the collarbone towards the shoulders.

STEP 4 KNUCKLING

Curl your hands into loose fists and place them palms down onto your lover's body. Work all over the chest making gentle circular movements with your fists.

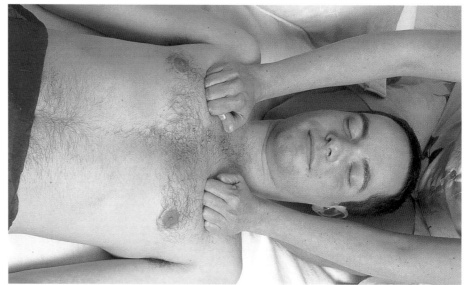

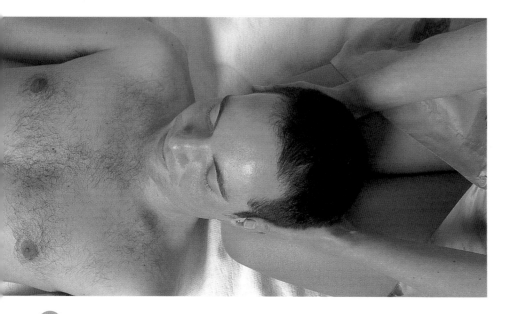

STEP 5 RELEASING NECK TENSION

Cup your hands around the back of the neck. Very gently and slowly, pull up the muscles of the neck using both hands at the same time.

STEP 6 SIDE STROKING THE NECK

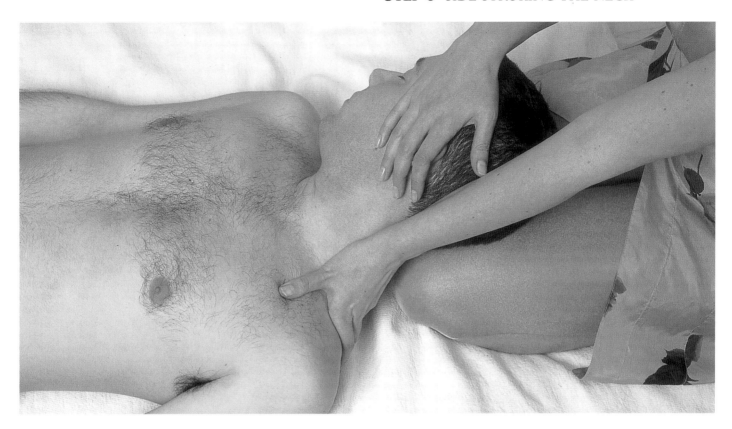

Turn the head to one side and place both hands at the base of the skull. Stroke down the neck with one hand and as it reaches the shoulder, follow it with the other hand.

STEP 7 THE FINAL TOUCH — BACK OF THE HAND STROKING OF THE CHEST AND NECK

Place the back of the hands gently down in the center of the chest. Barely touching your lover, stroke your fingertips out across the chest. Then use the back of your hands to fingertip stroke down the neck.

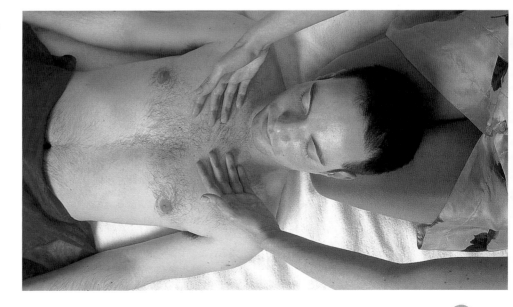

SENSUAL FACE MASSAGE

Massage of the face is a very intimate and sensual experience. It is also very rejuvenating and can make you and your lover look years younger as lines caused by stress and tension are reduced and the complexion takes on a healthy glow.

STEP 1 TUNING IN

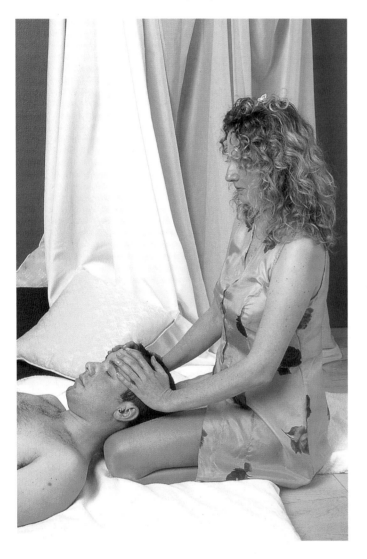

Lower your hands gently down onto your lover's forehead, and rest them there whilst you take a few deep breaths. Feel the worry and anxiety melting away.

STEP 2 STROKING THE FOREHEAD

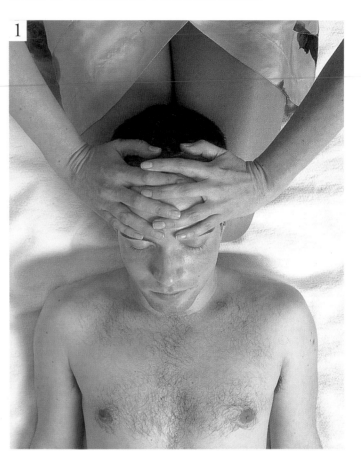

Stroke out across the forehead towards the temples and glide gently back with a feather light touch(1, 2). This movement is excellent for relieving headaches and tension.

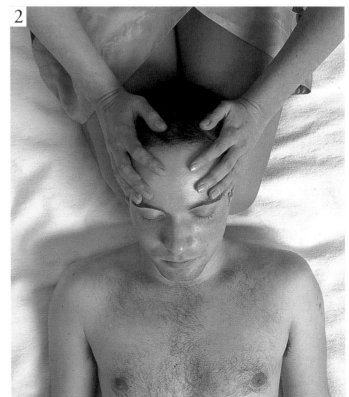

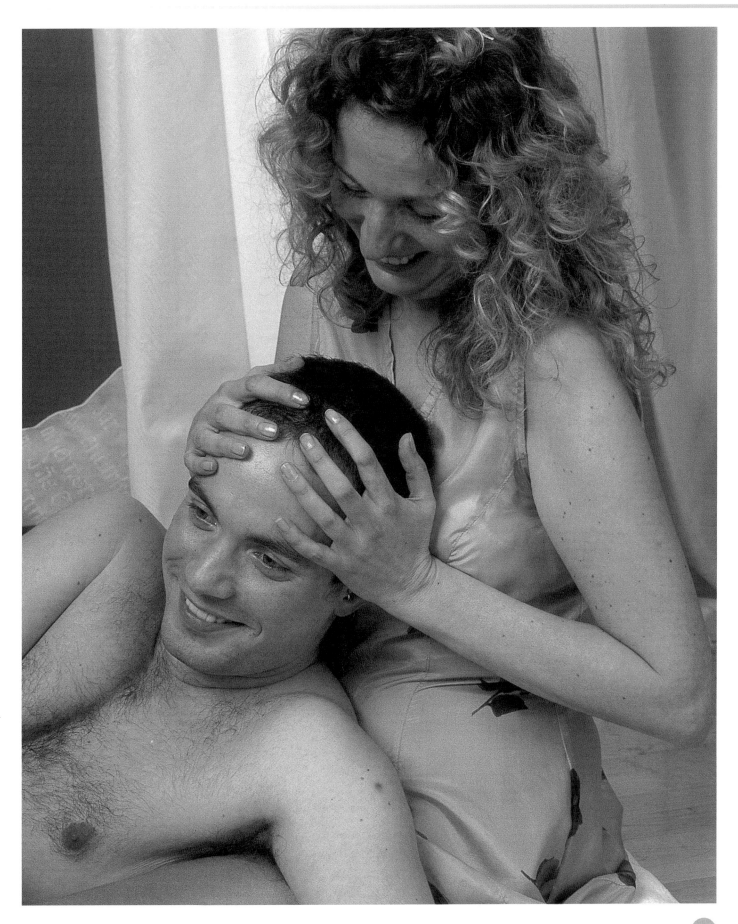

STEP 3 STROKING THE CHEEKS

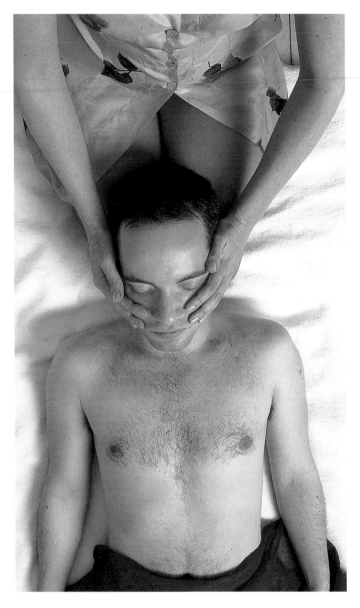

Using the fingertips and palms of your hands, stroke outwards across the cheeks and glide back again.

STEP 4 STROKING THE CHIN

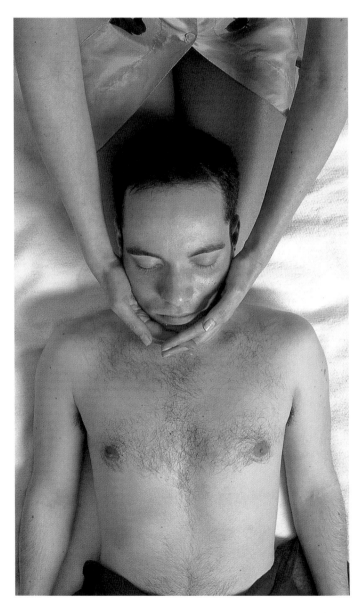

Stroke outwards across the chin and then continue stroking down the neck towards the shoulders.

STEP 5 PRESSURE CIRCLES ON THE FACE

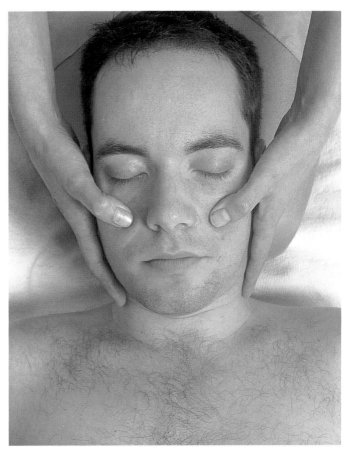

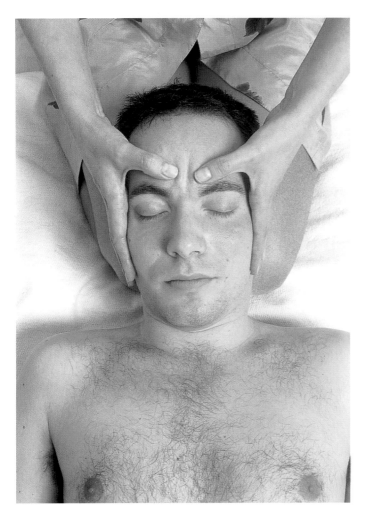

Lower your hands so that your thumbs come to rest just below the eyes. Repeat the gentle pressure circles in horizontal rows until you have completely covered the cheek area.

Place both thumbs in the center of the forehead just below the hairline. Using gentle pressure circles, work outwards across the forehead. After your first row, return your thumbs to the center of the forehead but move them down slightly. Repeat these rows until you reach the eyebrows.

Now place both thumbs in the center of the chin and repeat this technique to cover the entire chin and jaw area.

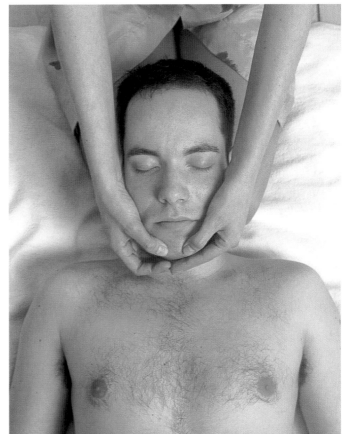

STEP 6 MASSAGING THE EARS

The ears are a very sensual area, and it is a delightful experience to have them massaged. Using your thumbs and forefingers, make small pressure circles all over the ears. Then stretch and release the ears very gently.

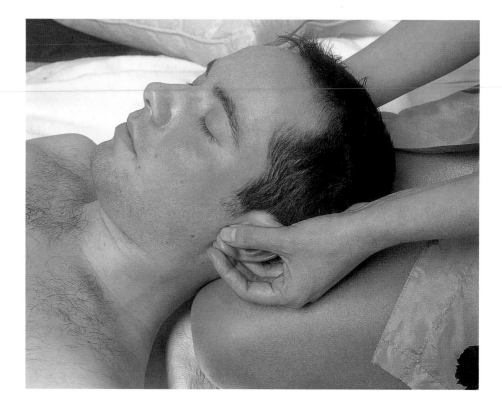

Stroke the hair and run your fingertips very gently through it to release any remaining tension in the head and scalp area.

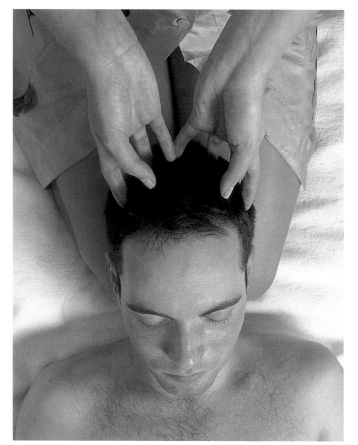

quick reference
Treatments

THE BACK

1. Tune in
2. Spreading the oil/long stroking
3. Alternate hands long stroking
4. Circle stroking
5. Stretching the back (hands)
6. Stretching the back (forearms)
7. Pulling up the sides of the back
8. Kneading the sides of the back
9. Circular thumb pressures on the spinal muscles
10. Pushing down the sides of the back
11. Circular stroking of the buttocks
12. Kneading the buttocks
13. Pressures on the sexual arousal points
14. Knuckling the buttocks
15. Plucking the buttocks
16. Circling both shoulder blades
17. Circular stroking of one shoulder
18. Thumb pressure around the shoulder blade

Repeat steps 17 — 18 on the other shoulder

19. Kneading the shoulders
20. Kneading the neck
21. Long stroking the whole back
22. Diagonal stroking
23. Cat stroking
24. Stroking with the back of the hands
25. The final touch — fingertip stroking

BACK OF THE LEG

1. Tune in
2. Long stroking (both legs)
3. Kneading the leg
4. Knuckling the thigh
5. Alternate heel of hand stroking up the back of the thigh
6. Plucking the thigh
7. The final touch — alternate fingertip stroking

Repeat steps 3 — 7 on the other leg

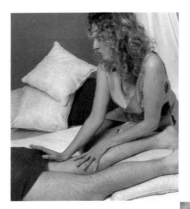

FRONT OF THE BODY

FOOT AND FRONT OF THE LEG

1. Greeting and stroking the foot
2. Kneading the foot
3. Spreading the foot
4. Push and pull the foot
5. Toe loosening
6. Freeing the ankle
7. Long stroking of the front of the leg
8. Kneading the thigh
9. Circular thumb pressures on the thigh
10. The final touch — fingertip stroking

Repeat all steps on the other foot and front of the leg

ARM AND HAND

1. Tuning in
2. Stroking the arm
3. Kneading the upper arm
4. Kneading the forearm
5. Loosening the wrist
6. Moving the wrist
7. Stroking the hands
8. Opening the hands
9. Stretch and squeeze the fingers and thumb
10. Circling
11. Fingertip stroking of the hand
12. The final touch — stroking of the arm

Repeat all steps on the other arm and hand

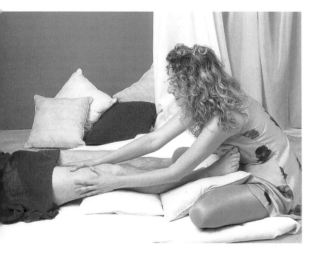

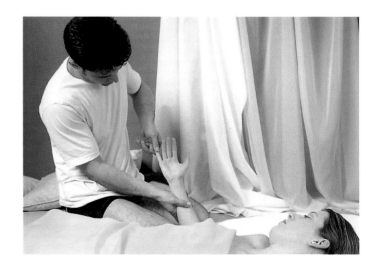

CHEST AND NECK

1. Tuning in
2. Opening up the chest
3. Circular pressures
4. Knuckling
5. Releasing neck tension
6. Side stroking the neck
7. The final touch — back of the hand stroking of the chest and neck

FACE

1. Tuning in
2. Stroking the forehead
3. Stroking the cheeks
4. Stroking the chin
5. Pressure circles on the face
6. Massaging the ears
7. The final touch — stroking the hair

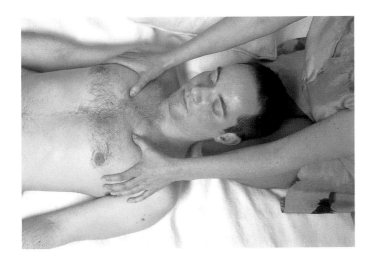

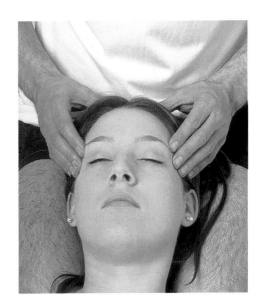

ABDOMEN

1. Tuning in
2. Circling the navel
3. Circle stroking
4. Pull
5. Kneading
6. The final touch — fingertip circular stroking

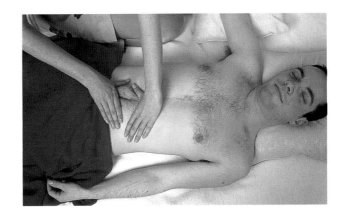

sensual massage for Common Problems

Making love should be a beautiful experience. However, problems can arise which interfere with our sexual enjoyment. This chapter explores how sensual massage and flower essences can help you to overcome any difficulties so that you can enjoy your sex life to the full.

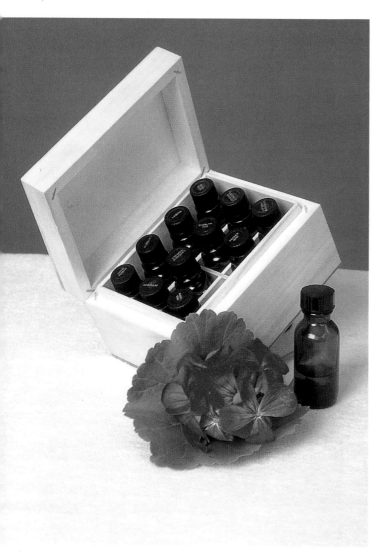

WOMEN

BREAST TONING

Women are never totally happy with the size of their breasts and it is unfortunate that to some it becomes an obsession. Usually women desire larger breasts and the following formulae may not increase size, but they will certainly help to tone the breasts and give them a more attractive appearance.

To two teaspoons of carrier oil add:
1 drop of geranium
1 drop of fennel
1 drop of clary sage

OR

To two teaspoons of carrier oil add:
1 drop of geranium
1 drop of lemongrass
1 drop of rose

Massage each breast outwards towards the underarms in a circular direction every day, and you should notice an improvement after a couple of months.

Geranium is an excellent oil for helping to tone the breasts.

INFERTILITY

Massage is very successful for treating women's infertility. Obviously if there is a serious physiological problem then it is unlikely that essential oils can succeed. However, there are many women who are unable to conceive for no reason at all.

Sensual massage is the perfect solution for relieving all the stress and anxiety which surrounds the longing for a baby.

The essential oil that seems to enjoy the most success is rose otto. Any of the formulae below can aid conception.
Massage them into the lower back (shown here) and abdomen daily. They should also be used as a prelude to making love when ovulation is due.

To two teaspoons of carrier oil add:
1 drop of rose otto
2 drops of geranium

OR
To two teaspoons of carrier oil add:

2 drops of clary sage
1 drop of melissa

Gentle massage of the lower back is an effective way to aid fertility in women.

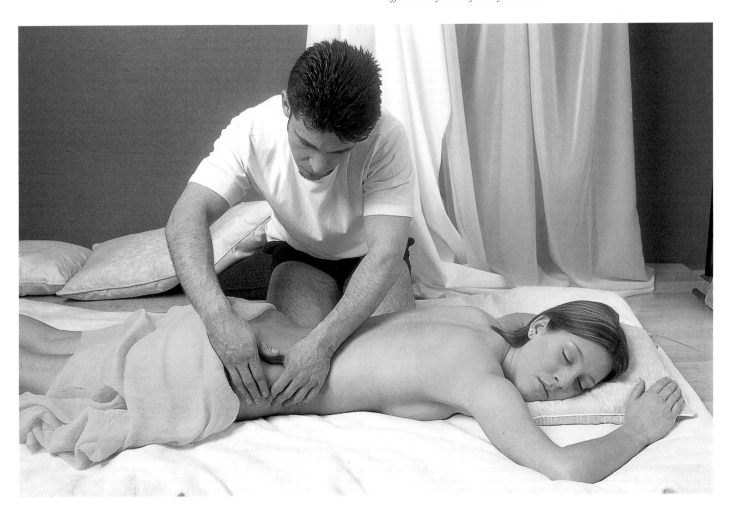

LOW SEX DRIVE

Whether you wish to increase your libido or you have an aversion to sexual intercourse, sensual massage is beneficial. Tiredness and anxiety due to work pressures and family or money worries will deplete any woman's sex drive. Women who are bored or left unsatisfied will also have a poor sexual appetite.

Sensual massage used alone will boost libido but when combined with one or several of the erotic oils, is more powerful. Remember that the aromas you like best will be particularly effective. Some of the most effective oils for increasing desire in women are bergamot, clary sage, frankincense, jasmine, myrtle, neroli, patchouli, rose, sandalwood and ylang ylang.

Any of the erotic oils can be used daily in your bath. One of the following blends should be applied for at least two weeks paying particular attention to the thighs, abdomen, lower back and buttocks to ensure that all the sexual arousal points are stimulated.

To 10 mls (two teaspoons) of carrier oil add:
2 drops of bergamot
1 drop of neroli

OR

To 10 mls (two teaspoons) of carrier oil add:
2 drops of myrtle
1 drop of rose

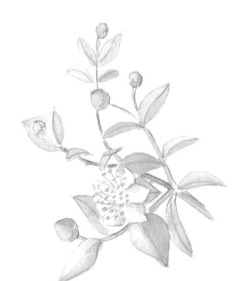

Myrtle and ylang ylang are just two of the essential oils used to boost libido.

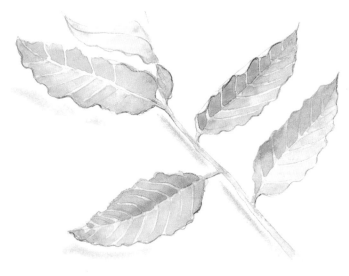

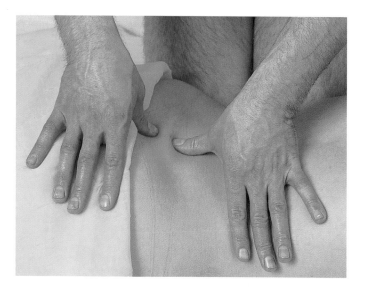

To raise a low sex drive, massage of the sexual pressure points, such as those situated on the lower back and buttocks, can be very effective.

VAGINAL DRYNESS

Lack of vaginal secretion makes intercourse uncomfortable or even impossible. It is not usually caused by a woman finding her lover unattractive. Anxiety, the menopause, or the contraceptive pill are far more likely to be the culprits.

Prior to intercourse, a small amount of jojoba carrier oil applied to the vagina is a temporary solution. However, daily baths or regular massage with one of the formulae will have a longer lasting effect.

Baths
3 drops of clary sage
2 drops of geranium
1 drop of rose

OR

1 drop of melissa
2 drops of neroli
3 drops of sandalwood

Massage
To 10 mls (two teaspoons) of carrier oil add:
1 drop of geranium
1 drop of neroli
1 drop of sandalwood

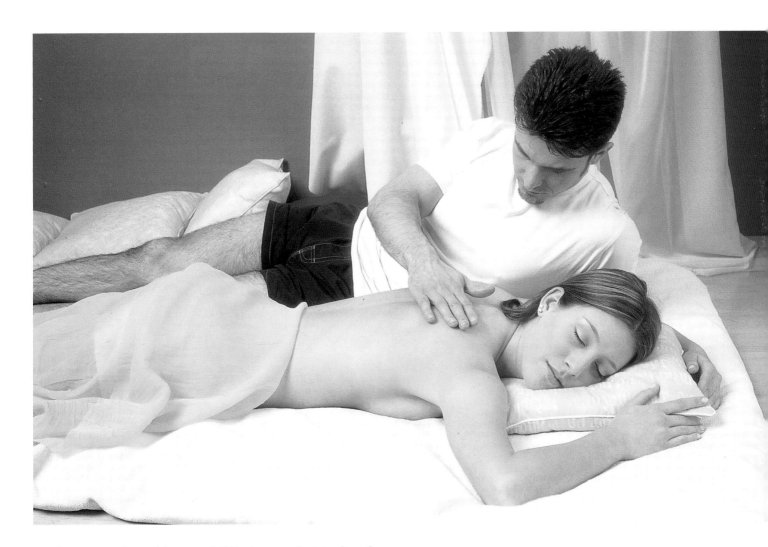

Regular massage with one of the suggested oil blends can ease feminine discomfort.

MEN

IMPOTENCE

Although drugs such as Viagra can improve your sex life, there will obviously be unwanted side effects. Sensual massage offers a natural alternative for boosting a man's sex drive.

Impotence is the most common male sexual disorder and it affects most men, often temporarily, at some point in their lives. Psychological factors such as stress, lack of confidence, guilt or depression can all lead to impotence. Physical illnesses such as diabetes can also be the cause, as can various drugs such as antidepressants, diuretics and blood pressure tablets.

A daily bath with one of the erotic essential oils is recommended. Suitable oils include black pepper, cedarwood, clary sage, frankincense, ginger, jasmine, neroli, rose, sandalwood and ylang ylang.

Sensual massage of the abdomen, thighs and back will also help with particular attention to the sexy stimulation points. Do not expect immediate results it may take two weeks or it may take two months.

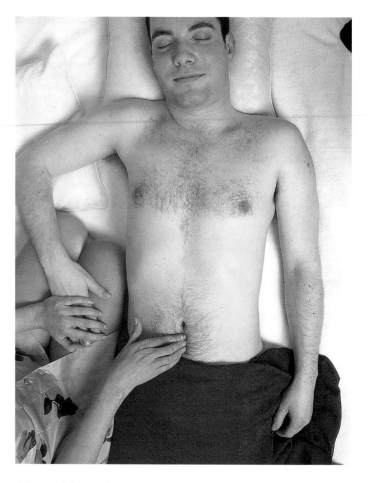

Massage of the sexual massge points, such as those on the abdomen can aid impotence.

To two teaspoons of carrier oil add:
1 drop of black pepper
1 drop of cedarwood
1 drop of ginger

OR

To two teaspoons of carrier oil add:
1 drop of neroli
1 drop of ginger
1 drop of sandalwood

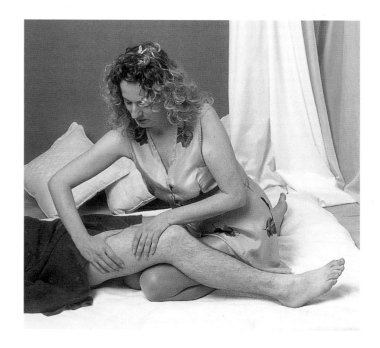

Another way to boost the male sex drive is sensual massage of the thighs.

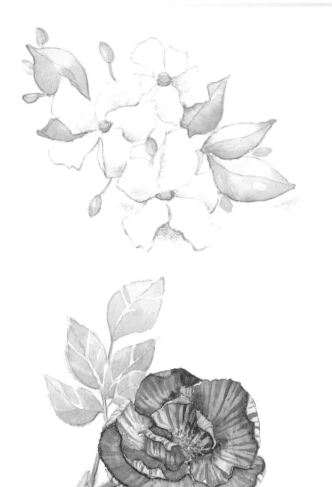

Jasmine and rose seem to be the most effective oils for increasing sperm count.

LOW SPERM COUNT

Both the quality and quantity of sperm is rapidly falling, and because of this male infertility is becoming more common. At the present time sperm defects are responsible for a quarter of all cases of infertility. However, fertility can be increased in the following ways.

1. There are several essential oils that may increase the sperm count. The most effective of these appear to be jasmine and rose. Make up a massage oil using two drops of jasmine and one drop of rose to 10 mls (two teaspoons) of carrier oil. Pay particular attention to the lower back area and the lower muscles of the abdomen to stimulate the production of sperm.

2. The optimum temperature for sperm production is 95°F, and if the testicles are too warm then the production of sperm is affected. Therefore men should avoid tight underwear, hot baths and saunas. Immersing the scrotum in cold water for at least ten minutes twice a day is also said to increase sperm production.

3. Smoking lowers both the quality and quantity of the sperm so stopping is vital.

4. Heavy drinkers have a low sperm count. Therefore men should not exceed more than 21 units per week.

5. Diets also have an important part to play. More fruit and vegetables (especially organic) are excellent, as are vitamins C and E, selenium and especially zinc.

6. Stress is also a contributory factor as it adversely affects the quality of semen. Regular sensual massage at least twice a week can significantly reduce it.

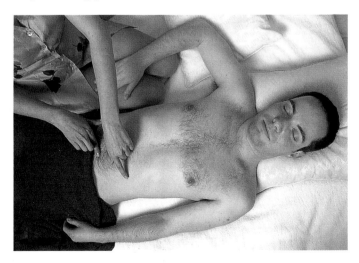

The lower abdomen contains sexual pressure points that can be stimulated to increase sperm count.

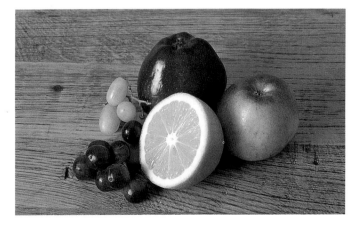

Diet also plays an important role in maintaining male fertility. Ensure that plenty of fresh fruit is eaten regularly.

flower
Remedies

Flower essences can help us to unlock our full potential and resolve our sexual difficulties. These remedies come from all corners of the globe and provide an excellent way to balance mind, body and spirit. Those remedies, which can help you overcome sexual difficulties are described here.

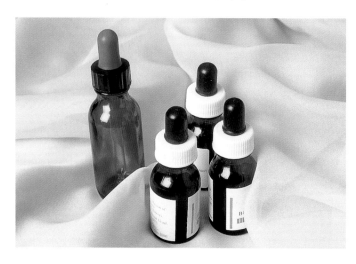

As well as the essential oils described in this book, there are a wide variety of Flower remedies from around the world that can be used to treat and ease problems and ailments.

MIXING A REMEDY

You will need a 30ml tinted dropper bottle, some spring water and a little brandy. Fill the dropper bottle almost to the top with spring water and add a teaspoon of brandy to preserve your remedy. You may use apple cider vinegar as a substitute for the brandy if you prefer. Put 2 drops of each of your chosen essences into the bottle.

HOW OFTEN TO TAKE THE REMEDY

Take seven drops three times a day either straight onto the tongue or in a glass of water, juice or herbal tea. The remedy should be administered for ten to fourteen days. In chronic cases they may need to be taken for a longer period.

ESSENCES FROM THE AUSTRALIAN BUSH

Australian aborigines have used flowers for thousands of years to heal the emotional and physical problems. Australia has the world's oldest and largest number of flowering plants. It is also one of the most unpolluted countries.

Billy Goat Plum

Useful for sexual revulsion or disgust of oneself. This remedy will enable you to relax and enjoy sex.

Flannel Flower

For those who have a dislike of being touched, particularly males. Flannel flower encourages sensitivity and sensuality.

She Oak

For infertility, particularly if there appears to be no reason.

Wisteria

For women who have a fear of intimacy, frigidity. Their fear may have arisen from sexual abuse. This remedy encourages a fulfilling sexual relationship.

ESSENCES FROM EUROPE — BACH FLOWER REMEDIES

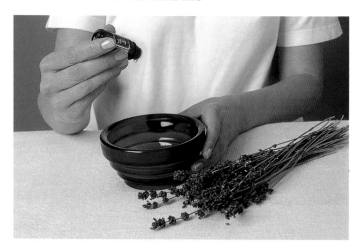

Crab Apple

For self-disgust. This is a remedy that helps to cleanse away traumas from the past, e.g. sexual abuse.

Larch

For boosting confidence and dispelling feelings of inadequacy. Excellent for problems such as premature ejaculation, impotence, and frigidity.

Olive

For tiredness and exhaustion. This remedy helps to boost libido.

Mimulus

For fear of failure, e.g. fear of premature ejaculation, fear of sex, fear of intimacy, etc

White Chestnut

For any sexual worries which circulate in the mind.

ESSENCES FROM INDIA

Cannon Ball Tree

For frigidity in women who are very fearful of sex.

Ixora

For couples who have lost sexual interest in each other. This remedy will enhance sexual activity.

Meenalih

For people who try to repress their sexuality as they have been brought up to believe it is sinful.

Rippy Hillox

For those who are fearful about sex due to a traumatic experience in the past, e.g. rape.

Water Lily

For anyone who is inhibited about sex.

NORTH AMERICAN FLOWER ESSENCES

Black-Eyed Susan

For those who have repressed traumatic sexual experiences such as rape or incest.

Easter Lily

For those who feel that sex is impure and unclean.

Hibiscus

For women who are unresponsive to sex — often due to prior sexual abuse.

Sticky Monkeyflower

For those who have a fear of sexual intimacy.

HAWAIIAN FLOWER ESSENCES

Amazon Swordplant

For those who need to break down their emotional blocks.

Avocado

For those who have a fear of being touched. This remedy promotes relaxation and sexual pleasure.

Day-Blooming Waterlily

For those who have a negative mental attitude towards sex due to feelings of fear, guilt, and inadequacy. This remedy encourages sexual fulfilment.

Lehua

For increasing sensuality in both men and women

Night Blooming Waterlily

For developing and enriching a close sexual relationship.

Spider Lily

For men who are afraid of relationships with women.

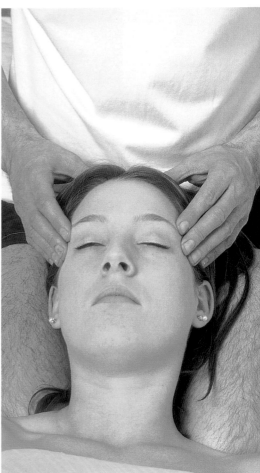

One drop of your chosen flower essence may be added to your massage blend to help to ease sexual problems.

Conclusion

You and your lover should by now have discovered the pleasures of both giving and receiving sensual massage and hopefully the experience has brought harmony, joy, and excitement to your relationship. You have probably by now created your own special massage movements for each other and developed your own love potions.

Regular sex is an important part of a long-term relationship. A 10-year study carried out by Dr. Weeks, a consultant neuro-psychologist of the Royal Edinburgh Hospital, reveals that couples who have sex at least three times a week look more than 10 years younger! Dr. Weeks interviewed more than 3,500 people aged 18-102 in Britain, Europe and the United States who were in established relationships to reach his conclusions. Therefore, if you practice sensual massage regularly not only is it highly pleasurable, but it is also excellent for your health and it makes you look more youthful!

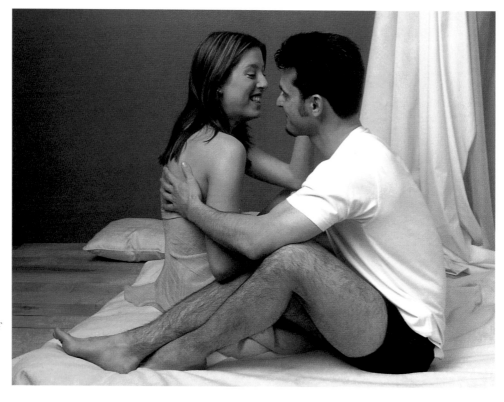

Both giving and receiving a sensual massage is an erotic experience for yourself and your lover. Hopefully you will feel relaxed, intimate and happy together.

Useful Addresses

UK
Beaumont College of Natural Medicine
Denise Whichello Brown
23 Hinton Road, Bournemouth
Dorset BH 2EF
(44)0202 708887

USA
American Massage Therapy Association
820 David Street
Suite 00
Evanston IL6020–4444
847/864–023

Index

Picture Credits:
Quarto Publishing, E.T. archive,
ACE Photo Agency

All other pictures © Quantum Books Ltd.

Many thanks to the models:
Adam, Paula and Bruno